W0113138

Self-Medication and Society

The question of recourse to self-medication arises at the intersection of two partly antagonistic discourses: that of the public authorities, who advocate the practice primarily for economic reasons, and that of health professionals, who condemn it for fear that it may pose a danger to health and dispossess the profession of expertise. This book examines the reality of self-medication in context and investigates the social treatment of the notion of autonomy ever present in the discourses promoting this practice.

Drawing on fieldwork conducted in France, the author examines the material, cognitive, symbolic and social dimensions of the recourse to self-medication, considering the motivations and practices of the subjects and what these reveal about their relationship with the medical institution, while addressing the question of open access to medicines – a subject of heated debate between the actors concerned on themes such as competence, knowledge and responsibility.

A rigorous analysis of the strategies adopted by individuals to manage the risks of medicines and increase their efficacy, *Self-Medication and Society* will appeal to sociologists and anthropologists with interests in health, illness, the body and medicine.

Sylvie Fainzang is a French medical anthropologist and Director of Research in the INSERM (Cermes3). She is the scientific coordinator of the international network MAAH (Medical Anthropology At Home), the editor-in-chief of the international Journal *Anthropologie & Santé*, and the author of several books on illness and medicines.

Routledge Studies in the Sociology of Health and Illness

Available titles include:

Self-Medication and Society

Mirages of autonomy

Sylvie Fainzang

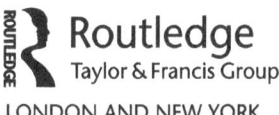

Routledge
Taylor & Francis Group

LONDON AND NEW YORK

First published 2017 by Routledge

2 Park Square, Milton Park, Abingdon, Oxfordshire OX14 4RN
52 Vanderbilt Avenue, New York, NY 10017

Routledge is an imprint of the Taylor & Francis Group, an informa business

First issued in paperback 2020

First published as *L'automédication ou les mirages de l'autonomie* by Presses Universitaires de France 2012

British Library Cataloguing-in-Publication Data
A catalogue record for this book is available from the British Library

Library of Congress Cataloging in Publication Data
Names: Fainzang, Sylvie, 1954- author.
Title: Self-medication and society : mirages of autonomy / Sylvie Fainzang.
Description: Milton Park, Abingdon, Oxon ; New York, NY : Routledge, 2017. | Series: Routledge studies in the sociology of health and illness | Includes bibliographical references and index.
Identifiers: LCCN 2016022088| ISBN 9781138213944 (hardback) | ISBN 9781315447162 (ebook)
Subjects: LCSH: Drugs—Prescribing. | Self medication—Social aspects. | Physician and patient. | Patient compliance—Social aspects.
Classification: LCC RM138 .F36 2017 | DDC 615.1—dc23
LC record available at https://lccn.loc.gov/2016022088

ISBN: 978-1-138-21394-4 (hbk)
ISBN: 978-0-367-59582-1 (pbk)

Typeset in Times New Roman PS
by diacriTech, Chennai

Table of contents

Acknowledgements

This book was first published in French by the Presses Universitaires de France in 2012, under the title *L'automédication ou les mirages de l'autonomie*, and was awarded the Prescrire 2013 Prize.

The translation was made by Jenefer Bonczyk and funded by the USPC (Université Sorbonne Paris Cité) programme 'The person in medicine'.

Introduction

The question of recourse to self-medication in France today arises at the intersection of two partly antagonistic discourses: that of the public authorities and that of health professionals. Recently advocated by the former mainly for economic reasons while condemned by the latter who fear it may pose a danger to health and dispossess them of their expertise, self-medication is problematic for patients who find themselves in a situation where they must learn new behaviour.

Self-medication has been the object of contrasting perceptions over time linked to the social, economic, therapeutic and cultural implications of the practice. A previous study of the social uses of medicines (Fainzang, 2001b) revealed that individuals' image of self-medication differed depending on their cultural and religious background (Fainzang, 2005). On this point, a stronger tendency was observed among certain groups to practice and, above all, value self-medication, while other groups tended to deny practicing it and disapprove of it. Thus, refusing or choosing to practice self-medication was shown to be a socially and culturally conditioned attitude. It became clear that in accordance with the values expressed within the family, self-medication takes on a different status depending on the social and cultural characteristics of individuals, leading some to advocate it while others reject it. In response to the medical discourse that tended to consider self-medication as a deviant practice and, as such, condemned it, a large number of patients self-medicated but with a feeling of committing a transgression towards medical authority and attempted to hide the practice from their doctor (Fainzang, 2015) in order to appear to behave as a 'good patient'.

In contrast, the French government today widely encourages individuals to practice self-medication, seeing this as an effective means of reducing public health costs. They have put in place various public policies (a decree authorising open access to medicines, making a certain number of proprietary drugs no longer eligible for reimbursement, etc.) with the intention of promoting self-medication. These incentive measures are accompanied by recommendations to users that set the boundaries of the practice and define the conditions. A section of the medical body supports these recommendations, notably through the 'Ten Commandments of Self-Medication' circulated on several websites aimed at the general public. In this new context, it is appropriate to investigate the conditions in which users today decide to self-medicate.

A discussion on self-medication requires a preliminary clarification of what is understood by this term and some attention to the difficulties that arise from using it. The literal meaning of self-medication is the act of deciding on one's own accord to consume medicines. Lecomte (1999) thinks that, in a larger sense, 'in reaction to discerning a health problem, self-medication involves making a self-diagnosis and treating oneself without medical advice' but, in a narrower sense, it is 'the acquisition of a product without a prescription that we call self-medication' (p. 49). Numerous works have however demonstrated that the choice of a medicine at a certain time can be the result of a previous prescription. Clearly, a medicine can be acquired through a prescription but consumed in a different context from that in which it was prescribed, either for another ailment, or at a different time: this is nevertheless self-medication. As such, Grand-Filaire (1992) thought that acts of self-medication were mainly imitative since they were inspired by previous prescriptions. Likewise, according to an enquiry presented to the Annual Conference of the French Society of Pharmacology (Laure, 1998), the medicines used in self-medication came, in a large majority of cases, from the remains of treatments previously prescribed by a GP, while 28 per cent were bought on the initiative of the subject alone.[1] Thus we should refute an overly restrictive vision of self-medication that does not take into account all the possible and uncontrolled uses of a prescription (acquiring the medicine for later, for someone else, etc.). Self-medication should be understood in a much wider way than simply as the non-prescribed use of a medicine. Molina (1988) goes as far as thinking that when patients ask their doctor to prescribe them a medicine they believe to be efficacious, it is in truth the patients who are self-prescribing through the intermediary of the doctor and with his/her endorsement. Equally, Van der Geest et al. (1996) consider every medication to be self-medication to a certain point in that the doctor does not administer the medicine him/herself and so cannot be sure that it will be taken as prescribed.

We will not however go to this extreme and will stay more in line with Buclin and Ammon's (2001) view that self-medication is defined as individual recourse to a medicine under one's own initiative. More precisely, self-medication will be considered here as the *act, for the subject, of consuming a medicine under ones' own initiative without consulting a doctor for the case in question, whether the medicine is already in the subject's possession or is procured for this effect (in a dispensary or from another person)*. The decision was made to limit this study to medicines derived from biomedicine.[2]

Autonomy and health

Such a reflection involves linking the question of self-medication with that of autonomy, a value that is experiencing exponential growth in contemporary society (Ehrenberg, 2009; Jouan and Laugier, 2009). However, what autonomy are we actually talking about when we discuss patient autonomy? In general and in common understanding, autonomy describes the capacity of a subject to decide for him/herself the rules that he/she will obey, and the capacity to act deriving from this capacity (Gillon, 1985). However, the meaning attributed to this term and its implications vary depending on the context.

Autonomy is most often invoked in the fields of disability and chronic disease, which in fact give rise to different questions, although zones of overlap do exist between these fields. In the disability sector, the notion of autonomy is literally envisaged as the antonym of dependence. Myriam Winance (2007) thus opposed the 'autonomous' person 'who decides and acts alone, without recourse to a helper', and the 'dependent' person 'who, as a result of an illness or an accident, is no longer capable of undertaking the various activities of daily life (activities that are physical, social, etc.) without relying on a helper' (p. 84).

In the history of the doctor–patient relationship, the valorisation of autonomy is a relatively recent social reality in France. It gained respectability when doctors realised that a necessary condition, if not for recovery but at least to prevent the disease getting worse, was that the patient takes responsibility for his/her care. This belief is expressed in the encouragements made to patients to take responsibility for a certain number of chronic diseases, where patient cooperation is essential for the treatment to work well.[3] The question of autonomy thus also gives rise to a reflection on the place of patients, their decisions on their treatment and on the necessity of their participation in their care. Autonomy then becomes synonymous with a capability to manage alone a treatment proposed by the medical institution. Sociology has indeed shown that the transition from acute to chronic fosters patient cooperation, and that it is in this cooperation zone that patient autonomy is generally envisaged.

Beyond the necessity of patient cooperation for strictly therapeutic ends, a person's autonomy is also widely affirmed today in the health domain for ethical ends. This demonstrates the growing desire of the different actors within this field to grant patients a part in the decision-making and to allow them to take some responsibility within the framework of their care managed by the medical institution.

The import of this value in the health domain reflects a more general culture of autonomy which is developing in the Western world as a joint result of the new situation engendered by renewed questioning of the medical world (Dodier, 2002), and of the introduction of Anglo-Saxon models where the emphasis is on patient empowerment. In this regard, Kleinman (2002) discusses autonomy and personal responsibility as values situated 'at the heart of the national American ideology'. Indeed, through their participation in the treatment of their chronic diseases, patients can assert their power in order to control the modalities of this treatment, as Eugeni (2011) shows for instance with dialysis patients. However, here the modifications made by the patients to the treatment are more associated with a desire to be more comfortable than to alter the therapy itself. This shift in meaning can be found in a document by a team of Quebecois researchers (Rodriguez del Barrio, 2006) entitled: *Autonomous Management of Medication in Mental Health*. The intention was to put services in place to allow users to 'reappropriate power', which 'notably manifests as the exercise of free and informed choice when decisions are made at crucial points in one's life. This involves the active participation of the person concerned in choosing the way in which services and help are provided in order to achieve personal aims and realise one's full potential' (p. 11). As we can see, it is a case here of participating in the decision-making, not making the decision itself. The notion of 'autonomous management of medication' implies the possibility for medication users to assert their points of view and to be 'associated' in the decisions concerning their medical treatment. It is more a matter of consenting to the decisions than actually deciding. At best, this autonomy consists of being able to say 'yes' or 'no' to treatment proposals made by others. The question of autonomy, associated with the self-management of chronic illness (Walger, 2009; Vincent *et al.*, 2010; Rogers, 2010), and studied through the intervention of 'the autonomy principle' on which the rules on consent are based, is thus reduced to the patient's capability to agree to or refuse the care proposed. On this point, Baszanger (2010) showed that the healthcare system is challenging the notion of autonomy as it is proposed in bioethics in that it forces the patient to be autonomous, and that this coercion (rather than opposing medical power) adds to the doctors' influence on the patients. Autonomy becomes a necessary condition in becoming the 'good patient' required by the health system.

Ultimately, the notion of autonomy is more often invoked either to valorise the patients' cooperation in their care package or to account for the freedom to consent or not to a treatment proposed by a doctor (Gagnon, 1995). The notion of 'decision-making power' is indeed always envisaged within the healthcare proposed by the medical institution. It is also within this framework that the notion of patient 'empowerment' is conceived, as the equivalent of 'decision-making power' through a deviation from its original meaning. Generally used to refer to the growth in the control patients have over political choices and over the exercise of their rights through their active participation (thus echoing the Foucauldian notion of 'self-governance'), patient empowerment, the objective of authentic health democracy,[4] is becoming reduced to the power to decide to accept or refuse a treatment proposed. Therapeutic education too is often reduced to teaching correct treatment observance: there is no patient education on self-governance since the focus is on adopting behaviour that conforms to prescriptions, in line with the principle of delegation. The majority of works extolling patient autonomy in fact deal with the way the patient receives and adheres to, or not, the treatment proposed. Hoerni (1991) thus assimilated autonomy into 'patient participation in the decision' concerning them.

Autonomy ends up signifying the right to consent or not to a treatment. However, the subjects can be led to take a decision altogether outside of medical care. While individual autonomy is at the heart of the ethical project contained in the law of 4 March 2002 (Orfali, 2003), the principle of autonomy tends to be confused with the principle of consent. Although it is a fundamental value in medical ethics (Faden and Beauchamp, 1986), autonomy in fact often refers to the patient's freedom when dealing with the doctor – with the doctor but not without him.

But up to what point do patients feel free to act without a doctor, in a way that is *emancipated* from medical authority? The question of patient autonomy is pertinent not only within the framework of care provision by doctors but also in the absence of a medical consultation. This is the case with self-medication. The anthropological dimension of self-medication largely resides in the fact that there is, with self-medication, a rupture in dependence on doctors. The question of knowing the conditions in which the subjects believe it appropriate to treat themselves relates to this rupture in dependence on medical authority. Alongside the ethical notion therefore emerges a political one.

Autonomy and self-medication

In this book I will examine the social treatment of the notion of autonomy within the framework of self-medication. The reflection will be more centred on the decision to take recourse to a medicine as a *practice* rather than the medicine as an *object* of medical technology, even though one can only be conceived in reference to the other. For a certain number of people, self-medication is today considered as a means of taking a greater responsibility for one's health; it is a case, for those using it, of affirming one's autonomy as regards one's health and one's independence vis-à-vis the doctors. Indeed, a CSA/Cecop[5] study into self-medication in 2007 (CSA/CECOP, 2007) revealed that 55 per cent of the respondents believed that self-medication amounts to 'autonomously managing one's health'. Self-medication is particularly appreciated by users who do not want to have to pass through professionals (doctors or even pharmacists), and see in it a means of freeing themselves from professional authority. And indeed, it is in the name of autonomy, and the moral and citizen categories such as responsibility that come with it, that self-medication is becoming more and more encouraged and advocated today.

However, what autonomy are we discussing in the case of self-medication? The aim of this work is to examine what takes place before, after or without the doctors, in other words, outside any encounter with them. Thus the reader is invited to a reversal of perspective, since it is not a case of the subject consenting to decisions but of deciding for him/herself on the treatment (be that medicinal) to be administered. As Thoer *et al.* (2008) underlined: 'the question of subject autonomy is at the centre of the practice of medicinal use outside medical advice and of the demands, expressed both individually and collectively by individuals, for a more immediate access to prescription drugs' (p. 37).

Here it is clearly not a case of examining the subject's autonomy within the autonomy/dependence dichotomy, nor in terms of patient participation, cooperation and consent. Instead it is examined in the sense of individual management of one's body and illness, since in self-medication users do not 'consent' to the care proposed but administer it themselves. Self-medication brings into play an autonomy where individuals decide on a treatment for themselves in accordance with their personal history, the information they possess about their affliction, what they identify as a symptom, their perception of the way health professionals have dealt with their problems in the past, etc. Thus we will attempt to focus more precisely on what is happening before, after or in the absence of medical prescriptions.

Self-medication is directly linked to the notion of autonomy by the very fact that recommending self-medication is an incitement to forgo, in some cases, the mediation of a medical prescriber. Recommending self-medication thus amounts to advocating that individuals take some of their healthcare in hand, in an autonomous way.[6] We will thus focus on what takes place outside of, or at a distance from, previous consultations to examine the conditions in which individuals choose to take recourse to self-medication. This point of departure entirely refutes Parsons' (1955) understanding of the ill person's role as one of submission to the doctor, since to the contrary, self-medication is tantamount to choosing to do without such an intervention. If the principle of autonomy valorises the subjects' capacity to decide for themselves, what are the driving forces behind their choices and decisions in terms of medicinal consumption? Is this autonomy effective? Is it valued by all segments of society? How, in actual fact, do patients enact their desire to be autonomous and apply the new instructions relating to their autonomy? From what point in time and in which situations is this autonomisation exercised or not? In other words, how do individuals experience and act upon this autonomy? The growing importance assigned to individuals in global society invites us to rethink the way in which the initiatives they take on the subjects of therapy and medical care provision are treated socially. But the public discourse on self-medication today also invites us to investigate the actual role of autonomy in this domain.

In an attempt to establish a classification in order to clarify the components of this notion, Gillon (1985) distinguished between (1) autonomy of action (which implies individuals are fully self-sufficient, that they are mobile for example); (2) autonomy of will (which corresponds to the possibility of self-determination, by virtue of which individuals can choose their course of action, without exterior influence or coercive pressure, after a personal deliberation and free from all contingencies); and (3) autonomy of thought (which requires knowledge, a critical mind, understanding, and a conscience to enable reflection).[7]

While the first form relates to autonomy as it is defined in the field of disability, the two other forms apply to the autonomy in question in the domain of self-medication.

Although, in a literal sense, the exercise of autonomy results from the fact of imposing laws on oneself – and the works on autonomy frequently remind us of its etymology: *auto-nomos* (*auto*: oneself; *nomos*: law) – and it describes the individual's right to freely determine the rules he/she follows (Schneider, 1998; Schneewind, 2001; Tristram Engelhardt, 2001), the autonomy of the subject practicing self-medication cannot for all that be exercised in a totally independent way, wholly outside of all exterior influences. As we will see, their choices are partly built and conditioned by advice from close family and friends, advertising, Internet consultation (either from recommendations published on professional sites or opinions expressed on discussion forums), etc. Individuals are never totally independent: they are exposed to a thousand influences from family, colleagues and friends as well as global society.[8] Although, at any mention of autonomy the focus tends to be on the individual, at least in Western societies,[9] the individual (patient, user, consumer, etc. – we will come back to the choice of terms) is never alone. As R. Massé (2003) remarked, the recognition of free will in decision-making does not imply 'a conception of a theoretical citizen who is totally free of exterior influences. Every one of us is influenced, even to a certain extent constrained, by the pressure of family members, by the values, norms, duties and obligations of society. (…) In fact, autonomy is always delineated and limited by diverse sources of credible and legitimate authority or, at least, by sources recognised as such by the individual' (p. 219).

But these latter only appear indirectly, since the subject is the sounding board for these different influences. Whether users follow a previous prescription or not, and whether they ask for advice from a pharmacist or not – this behaviour being only one aspect or one possible moment of their strategy – the emphasis in self-medication is squarely placed on the role of individuals, on their choices, and on the exercise of their autonomy.

The notion of Subject is better suited to accounting for the multiple influences exerted on the individual. Numerous authors have made statements on their choice of the term 'ill person' or 'user' in preference to 'patient' (see McLaughlin, 2009, concerning service–recipient relationships). Some criticise the commercial connotations contained in the notion of 'user', while others object to the idea of passiveness in the face of a doctor or medical institution inherent in the word 'patient'. 'Patient' implies one is subjected to a treatment or a care programme, even though the individual's role as an actor in the field of health is now recognised (Soum-Pouyalet, 2007; Van der Geest, 2010[10]). To summarise his distinction between 'ill person' and 'patient', Pierron (2007) wrote: 'we suggest that the subject is ill when he/she presents biological signals of which the symptomatologic depth affects his/her biography, whereas the subject is a patient when he/she agrees to lose the initiative as regards the illness, handing it to the doctor who provides a meaning to the symptom and proposes a therapeutic response' (2007: 50).

In truth, another difference exists between these words, to the point that they cannot be easily substituted for one another. This difference relates to a distinction between diverse experience regimes and social statuses. The term 'ill person' describes the state of the subject vis-à-vis the illness (involving the state of his/ her body) while the word 'patient' describes the state of the subject vis-à-vis the institution to which he/she turns and the person representing it. While 'ill person' denotes the state of the subject without presupposing any care, the word 'patient' includes him/her *de facto* in a relationship with a care provider. The first places the subject in relation to the illness, the second in relation to the doctor. The first situates the subject outside the doctor–patient relationship, the second on the contrary integrates the subject into the relationship. Therefore we cannot use the word 'patient' to designate the position of the person practising self-medication since strictly speaking, in the act of self-medication, the subject does not take recourse to a medical institution and does not enter into a medical relationship. The use of the word 'patient' in the texts pertaining to self-medication (notably in Academie nationale de pharmacie, 2006 and in Coulomb and Baumelou, 2007) is thus not appropriate. In the case of self-medication, the person does not rely on medical authority but actively decides on the medicinal treatments to take. The subjects in question are resolutely not *patients* since they are perceived here to be operating outside any intervention by a doctor. With self-medication, it is the subjects who give a meaning to their symptoms and who provide the therapeutic response. Here, it is precisely their status as active beings – actors capable of making choices and taking decisions – that is at stake. Yet, using the term 'ill person' is problematic as the subjects may not necessarily think of themselves as 'ill' at the time they choose to medicate. The most pertinent term would be 'subject' when discussing the position of autonomy inherent in self-medication, in other words, when making reference to individuals who consider themselves to be ill at a given time, or who are experiencing a disorder, or even who would like to prevent an illness, which leads them to take medicines of their own accord and become users. Using the term 'subject' does not mean patients are considered as passive beings, totally devoid of their role as actors as highlighted in the social sciences, but nor does it mean they are considered to be totally independent. In proposing this conceptualisation of the term 'subject', I aim to make reference to the character of the individual as both acted-upon and acting, i.e. to the partly chosen and partly imposed role that the individual plays. Individuals are *Subjects* as the *subject of the verb* is, they are the author and sometimes the master of their acts; but they are also subjects as a *subject of the king* might be, meaning partly subservient or subjugated to a power beyond their own, in this case the social determinants, the political context and the cultural influences – in other words, to laws and rules other than their own. The subjects' dependence on social structures and their relative submission to cultural influences does not invalidate the portion of choice left to them.

On this point, we should note the imprecise way in which the term 'family medication' is sometimes used in lieu of 'self-medication'. This is notably the case in a press release from cabinet ministers concerning the publication of a report entitled '*Situation de l'automédication en France et perspectives d'évolution*' ('The situation of self-medication in France and the outlook for the future').[11] Yet, it is important to differentiate between the notion of 'family medication' and that of 'self-medication'. Strictly speaking, we cannot assimilate these two notions, even if these practices sometimes overlap and in both cases a decision is made to medicate without medical advice. In the first term the emphasis is on the role of the family (the domestic choices as opposed to expert decisions), while in the second there is the idea of personal choice, which does not place the users in the same position in terms of how their rights are exercised. Individual opinions are not necessarily in line with those of other family members and the individual dimension of the act, which disappears under the collective notion of the 'family', is an important part of self-medication. The use of one term or the other entails very different economic, symbolic and social implications.

In all of this, the result is that an investigation into the question of autonomy in the field of self-medication involves examining not so much the relationship to medicines taken as self-medication but the relationship to the very *practice* of self-medication. This is why this book focuses less on medicines as therapeutic objects or products of a medical technology, and more on self-medication as a social behaviour (Nichter and Vuckovic, 1994; Whyte, Van der Geest and Hardon, 2002). This perspective takes a political rather than a technical approach to the act of self-medication. Thus I will take an interest in the subjects' decisions to take recourse to medicines (previously prescribed or not) of their own personal initiative, and endeavour to understand the mechanisms, motivations (be they practical, economic, philosophical or cultural), obstacles, modalities and temporalities involved.

Related questions

Within the framework of this study I will address a certain number of questions – either because they are inherent to the practice of self-medication, or because they are raised on a regular basis in the public space on this subject.

On this point, nourished by the debate surrounding the more general practice of self-medication and legalised in France by the decree of 30 June 2008, the subject of *open access* to medicines has caused much controversy. The actors concerned – the public authorities, industry, doctors, pharmacists and users – have staked out their positions and constructed their opposing discourses, of which I will examine the stakes and logics. They resort to arguments that correspond with the different interests motivating them (economic, therapeutic, professional, philosophical or political). All these arguments are based – although in different ways – on a rhetoric of responsibility and autonomy of which I will examine the meaning, impact and limits.

Anthropologists have comprehensively demonstrated that the way in which individuals perceive their ailment has an impact on their treatment pathways: the type of institution called upon, the choice of medicine used (biomedicine *versus* alternative medicines), or the order of the actions undertaken within their therapeutic itineraries. But the appearance or identification of a symptom does not necessarily result in a consultation with a health professional, since it could equally lead to self-medication. This course of action involves two principle operations: firstly, considering oneself to be ill or to be presenting a disorder susceptible to being cured by a medicine, and secondly, choosing to manage the problem oneself by medicinal means. The question is then one of discovering the conditions in which subjects identify a corporal event as pathological (even if their state of health is not serious or not likely to be given a nosological label validated by biomedicine), and the conditions in which they decide to self-medicate when confronted with a symptom. Recourse to self-medication entails adopting satellite behaviours such as clinical self-examination and self-diagnosis. It should be clarified that in epistemological terms a physical symptom is only relevant to our study when the subjects recognise it as such. If a subject has a fever but pays no attention to it and takes no action to address it, we would be dealing with something that may well be a symptom for a doctor but not necessarily for the subject, in the sense that he/she does not make it exist and does not manage it as such. In such a case, the situation will not be recorded within the framework of this study in that it does not lead to specific social or therapeutic practices. The anthropologist here only gives symptoms a reality if the subjects themselves acknowledge them. An individual not acknowledging a bodily phenomenon could of course interest an anthropologist in that it may be an expression of a denial which could be socially analysed or it may result from a cognitive schema where there is no place for the phenomenon. Almost all facts can come under an anthropological gaze, as long as they are the object of a pertinent and appropriate problematisation. Within the framework of this study, the prerequisite for a bodily sign to become a relevant fact is that the subject uses it as a reason to take recourse to self-medication. In conformity with the emic posture of anthropology, the symptoms discussed are therefore those that the subjects recognise as such.

The question of the role played by symptoms partly ties in with that of the opposition between the normal and the pathological, dear to studies on the construction of illness. However, it should be raised here in a different way. It is not enough to simply identify what the subjects perceive to be pathological to define the point at which they consider it necessary to consult a doctor or seek healthcare facilities; it is a question of discovering what makes the symptom suitable for recourse to self-medication *rather than* recourse to a professional and thus determining where the subjects believe the boundary lies between a pathological symptom that can be *self-managed* and a pathological symptom that should be dealt with by a professional or an institution. The examination of these questions will lead me to put certain categories of medical semiology to test on the ground. What are the motivations of, and the conditions for, a recourse to self-medication induced by the identification of a symptom? Many studies postulate pain or discomfort (for example loss of sleep) − symptoms that handicap the individual's daily life and work − as major reasons for self-medication. The ill person considers him/herself capable of making a diagnosis and of knowing what is needed to manage the affliction. It is commonly thought that it is often the inability to manage a bothersome or painful symptom through self-medication that leads to a consultation with a doctor. Yet, as we will see, the opposite can sometimes occur. This phenomenon demonstrates the degree to which the relationship with the medical institution is implicated in recourse to self-medication. In this regard, I will include the subjects' past experiences in order to put this practice into perspective and investigate its meaning.

The debate that rages around self-medication in the public space, as well as in the professional sphere, relates to a great extent to the question of competence. Are the transformations undergone in the status of ill people today, and in particular the strong emergence of a new 'patient power' (Rabeharisoa and Callon, 1999) which was the aim of the law dealing specifically with their rights (Law of 4 March 2002), still based on the recognition of knowledge? And what knowledge is this? Here I will use several different situations to examine the constitution and development of individual knowledge but also the associated pitfalls, in order to show how knowledge is a fundamental stake both in the social debate on the competence of ill people and in their recourse to self-medication.

The question of the risk inherent in this practice hinges on that of individual competence and capability in self-medication. On this point, we should clarify that the public authorities only encourage self-medication in 'benign situations' (as is made clear on the ministry of Health website).[12] But how do subjects distinguish between benign and non-benign situations? This assessment depends both on the individual's history and on the cognitive logics at work in the practice of self-medication. The subjects should first assess, in a responsible way, the appropriateness of using self-medication or consulting a doctor. Consequently, they should be capable of evaluating the risks and the efficacy of the decision, the risk being that in deferring recourse to a professional, a delay in diagnosis could damage their health. But there is also the risk of medicinal misuse. These are the aspects that alarm the doctors. It is because of the danger represented on one hand by not consulting a doctor in time, and on the other by an inappropriate use of a medicine, that many health professionals are reluctant to support self-medication, even for benign pathologies. The risk being not only that the diagnosis could be wrong, but also that the medicines are unsuitable or badly used (Rose, 2005). The subjects however are fully aware of this danger and they develop a certain number of strategies that aim to reduce the risks associated with taking the medicines. In these conditions, how do the subjects manage this risk? How do they respond to the safety requirements of medicinal use? But also, what logics underpin the search for efficacy associated with the choice to 'self-medicate', given that it is precisely the efficacy of a substance that gives it the potential to carry risk?

By studying all these questions, I will thus examine the place of autonomy – how it is enacted and how it is treated socially – in the field of self-medication, in order to define its conditions and its limits within a process I will qualify as 'self-medicalisation'.

Methodology

I met the forty or so informants who participated in this study mainly through the so-called 'snowball' method. The first informants, who matched the population chosen for the study, indicated other potential informants through their interknowledge networks (friends, family members, work colleagues, association members, etc.), who in turn designated people they knew, who were added to the sample group constituted in this way. This method allowed me to approach a relatively varied population. In choosing this mode of inclusion I did not in any way aim to form a representative sample of the population (this in fact is not the ambition of anthropology), at least in the statistical understanding of the idea of representativeness. This study does not claim to provide statistically representative results; instead it aims to discover certain mechanisms at work in recourse to self-medication. In the same vein as Marcel Mauss (1966) who claimed that 'it is an error to believe that the credit to which a scientific proposition is due depends narrowly on the number of cases with which it can be verified' (p. 391), Hamel (1998) distinguished between 'statistical representativeness' and 'theoretical representativeness'. He believes that the sample should be built by using what he calls 'methodological imagination' (Hamel, 2000) which endeavours to insure that the case studied presents episte-mological qualities that allow it to 'represent' the group and authorise generalisa-tion. As Bourdieu (1993) wrote: 'a well-built particular case ceases to be particular' (p. 57). A distinction is thus made between the object of the study (a given cultural group) and the group of informants that represent it and serve as an observatory.

Considering the statistically non-representative nature of the sample, the risk of reflecting a group that would be too socially homogenous has been partly miti-gated by the diversity of the interknowledge networks mobilised: some designated colleagues, others friends, others neighbours, etc., who in the end proved to be very different from the first informants (in their social, economic, ideological positions, etc.). By constructing a group of informants through personal connec-tions, we move further away, in the same movement and paradoxically, from the first type of people studied. Moreover, to limit this risk, I chose to multiply the departure points of the network, fostering the constitution of what could be con-sidered as a plurality of 'snowballs', each of the first flakes originating on differ-ent paths. Finally, this process reduced the difficulty of gaining access to people to discuss an object as personal and intimate as the treatment of one's body and illness, without having to pass through the intermediary of health professionals.

The inquiries were carried out at people's homes and consisted for a large part of interviews. This allowed me to gather a good number of accounts regarding pathological episodes, in order to bring to light different scenarios of self-medicinal use. We cannot however delude ourselves as to how much interviews alone can provide without being associated with an observation of actual practice. I can accurately determine these limits having relied heavily on observation in previous studies. Personal accounts are limited in that they are recounted by the subjects and are thus mediated by their memory, their awareness and their words. For its part, ethnographic observation of actions on the ground provides information that cannot be produced by a simple account of the past. This is not only because recounting an episode reduces its contents, but also because the subjects are not necessarily conscious of their actions or the mechanisms at work in their reason-ing and in their decision-making (such as the parameters according to which the choice to self-medicate and the practice of self-medication depend), nor the inter-est this could have for the study. Therefore, alongside gathering accounts, I carried out in situ observation, when possible,[13] of what the subjects chose to do when faced with a symptom.

The interviews dealt with established facts. A technique frequently used in quantitative studies on self-medication is to question informants on how they intend to behave in a hypothetical pathological or symptomatological situation. But this is an abstract situation, from which reality cannot be inferred. In this regard, an interview that aims to only ask questions such as 'What do you do when you are ill?', as many questionnaire-based studies do, does not provide much more information than asking the subjects: 'What would you do if you were ill?' or 'In what circumstances would you decide to self-medicate if you were ill?' The interview should relocate the practice of self-medication in its context, and make reference to lived events (past or present). In contrast with a study that relies on the 'intentional', it seemed preferable to study practices that have already been accomplished when they cannot be observed actually taking place. The past provides more information than the conditional.

Hence the need to see the informants several times over the long term, even if this involved asking them to repeatedly retell the story of their illness, and to incite comments to support the observed practices. Thus, the data was gathered by observing and interviewing people who believed they had in the past, or believe they currently have, an illness or health problem to resolve. It was thus necessary to go beyond the stage of questioning people on their practices of self-medication and the factors that led them there and to invite them to recount, based on concrete episodes of illness, the way in which they managed them. The stories of illness were often 'stories of symptoms' that led to recourse to self-medication, either exclusively or in association with another strategy. The accounts of self-medication in fact included different types of possible itinerary: some people first tried self-medication then went to a health professional (a GP or specialist), while others first went to a health professional before trying to self-medicate, some chose to do both simultaneously, while others again ended up returning to the first recourse after having tried the second, not to mention alternative or exclusive recourse to generalists or specialists. As far as possible, I tried to record the 'episodes' of illness and the types of reaction induced by the appearance or the reappearance of a symptom, and the conditions of and reasons for the decisions taken.

To partly mitigate the limits of the interview format compared to the unrivalled contribution of direct observation, I also sought to gain access to the informants' medicine cabinets, a method proven during a former research project on the relationship with medicines (Fainzang, 2001b). I sought to gather information on the conditions in which the medicines kept in the informants' domestic pharmacies were acquired in order to obtain complementary material. In addition, I gathered material on the views expressed by Internet users on the question of open access to medicines, the object of a controversy that I will examine further in this work.

The social sciences have highlighted the degree to which the social environment exercises an influence on health-related behaviour. The impact of social, cultural and economic factors on health-related behaviour in general is such that these factors must surely also have an influence within the framework of self-medication. The works on this subject (Barthe, 1990; Aïach and Cèbe, 1991; Raynaud, 2008) have thus shown that recourses to self-medication are largely constructed by the social environment to which the individuals belong. However, as we will see, the results of their studies diverge greatly. Therefore, it seems very hazardous to paint a sociological picture of the Subject of self-medication. Furthermore, if we take into account the great professional mobility of individuals (a huge phenomenon in these times of precarity) and the fact that some of the episodes reported took place when the person was working in a different profession from when discussing it, but also the growing gap between professional, economic and cultural statuses, it should be recognised that the respondents' socio-professional affiliation is not an element that always makes sense in understanding the materials gathered. So, when I provide such information, the reader will sometimes be surprised by the dissonance between the profession of the informant and the behaviours and opinions reported. Nevertheless, in order to define the mechanisms of self-medication that transcend the particularities built by contextual sociodemographic or socio-cultural data, I chose to confine the study to the vast contemporary category of 'the middle classes' (upper and lower, old and new)[14] in order to smooth out the contrast that overly heterogeneous social affiliations would offer or produce.

Beyond their social differences, the subjects' behaviours are also likely to vary in relation to the geographic accessibility of healthcare centres. This is why I tried to neutralise the potential effect of differing availability in care services on recourse to self-medication by only including people living in Paris and its inner suburbs, who were consequently placed in almost identical conditions in terms of geographical access to healthcare centres.

To carry out such a study, it was appropriate to not assume a position as a professional or an expert, which could have led the subjects to adopt behaviours they thought they should, or even to invent a discourse of a 'good patient'. While this position has proved productive, it also has its downsides. The subjects sometimes let themselves assume a position of expertise acquired through their experience and, armed with such knowledge, urged the anthropologist to forgo doctors and practise self-medication, and then provided advice on the subject.[15]

This type of research cannot avoid a whole series of difficulties linked to how the informants perceive the objective of the study itself, the image they have of it and the meaning they give it. The material collected from comments the subjects made in front of their medicine cabinets sometimes did not match with the data from the statements they made during the first interviews, either because they wanted to appear to conform to what they considered socially acceptable, or because of an oversight. For example, many people take hypnotics but did not report these as medicines taken through self-medication even though they were obtained from family members and administered without medical advice. Such consumption was often not mentioned during the interview but discovered when the person commented on the contents of their domestic pharmacy. Moreover, some acts were not reported as self-medication simply because the medicine had at one point in time been prescribed by a doctor. In this case, repeating the treatment in a later or different context did not necessarily make it an act of self-medication in the subjects' eyes.[16] Finally, some said they did not consume psychoactive drugs by self-medication simply because they did not know that the medicine they were taking fell into this category of drugs.

Another difficulty resided in trying to avoid using certain terms, phrases or key words in front of the informants. It was thus necessary to question each word and consider the effect its use may have. This difficulty is a constant in research where the use of certain terms, which may sometimes be key in that they constitute the very object of the research, can carry what could be perceived as a value judgement. The word 'self-medication' itself is very heavily charged because of the negative image it carried for a long time in France, especially when used by health professionals. In this regard, the interviews were as unstructured as possible in order to avoid inducing any particular response. For example, asking someone whether they sometimes borrow medicines from family or friends is from the outset a line of questioning that could appear to be marred by a judgement, and it risks heading towards a negative answer. Likewise, it is problematic to ask someone if he/she has ever postponed consulting a doctor. The notion of 'patient delay', often used to refer to a postponement in seeking treatment, and on which Sand Andersen (2010) carried out research, can be perceived to designate a negative behaviour or one likely to harm ones' health. The simple use of this term can be enough to let the subjects think the inquirer somehow disapproves. As if postponing a consultation necessarily implies a delay in diagnosis and consequently that the patient is responsible for the potential aggravation of the affliction.

Finally, this study included an emotional element that became evident when people discussed their illnesses and suffering. Even if pain is difficult to voice and communicate,[17] the person evoking it sometimes communicated distress that was difficult not to be moved by. From this empathetic posture, analytical detachment allowed me to distance myself, and all the more easily when the people themselves could be encouraged to describe, distance themselves from and interpret their own perceptions and practices.

In addressing all these questions, we will see that self-medication is a choice object for the anthropologist, despite the fact that it is disconnected, in the literal sense, from the doctor–patient relationship. Indeed, the individual here is dealt with individually and the social relationship thus appears to be excluded. Nevertheless, the act in question is very much socially constructed. But it is what self-medication also tells us, implicitly, about the relationship with the Other that makes it a true anthropological object. Self-medication reveals something about the doctor–patient relationship in the very absence of this relationship and maybe even precisely because of the refusal to include it in resolving one's experience.

Notes

English sentences cited in this text from publications in French are the author's translation.

1 The data on self-medication based on dispensary sales figures should however be treated with much caution. We cannot in fact rely solely on sales figures to accurately evaluate the real consumption of medicines taken through self-medication, because some medicines are bought, whether they are prescribed or not, and are not consumed (Fainzang, 2001b).

2 In contrast to many anthropological works that very often consider self-medication as a recourse to complementary or 'indigenous' medicines as opposed to biomedical technology (Lock and Nguyen, 2010), this research will exclusively address the practice of self-medicating industrial pharmaceutical products derived from biomedicine, even if this can be integrated into practices that borrow from heterodox belief systems.

3 This cooperation is deemed essential for diabetics for example who need to measure their insulin levels, or for people suffering from a respiratory disease who may be asked to measure their breathing using a peak flow meter (a device that monitors respiratory flow) in order to regulate their own medicinal doses in accordance with the level indicated by the test.

4 This very notion reflects the social objectives at the heart of the law concerning patient rights of March 2002.

5 Institut d'Etudes et de Conseil/Centre d'études et de connaissances sur l'opinion publique.

6 It should be noted that the public authorities, for their part, condemn and sanction the personal and autonomous decision to consult a specialist: it is now obligatory in France to pass by the intermediary of a GP in order to see a specialist.

7 A classification that has been partly taken on by the French National Consultative Ethics Committee for Health and Life Sciences (CCNE, 2005) in the reflection they undertook in order to give an opinion on treatment refusal.

8 Although in return, patient autonomisation is one of the results of the developments in information technologies since the Internet stimulates the growth of 'self-care' (Romeyer, 2008).

9 Autonomy is not always 'individual'; other societies do not perceive it as being dissociated from the family (we will return to this point).

10 'The term 'patient' is itself a symbol of the passive and powerless position of people who face health or disability problems' (Van der Geest, 2010, p. 98).

11 This press release revealed that 'Alain Coulomb, former director of the National Authority for Health and Professor Alain Baumelou, have today submitted their report on family medication to Xavier Bertrand, the minister for Health and Solidarity' (www.sante.gouv.fr).

12 www.sante.gouv.fr

13 Even though it is not always easy to observe, on the spot, people's actual gestures and acts.

14 See Chauvel (2006) on this subject.

15 Véronique, a French teacher, went the furthest. The interview finished with a 'consultation' where she searched for my 'aura' (a sort of halo supposed to glow around the body, only visible to the initiated, and which is the manifestation of an energy field or a life-force in the discourse of the occult sciences and some spiritual movements), and using this she tried to uncover a health problem.

16 For example, a woman regularly gives her child a cortisone-derived anti-inflammatory on her own initiative because a doctor once prescribed it to her, but she does not consider this act to be self-medication.

17 In her essay entitled, 'On being ill', Virginia Woolf deplores the paucity of language in this regard: 'but let a sufferer try to describe a pain in his head to a doctor and language at once runs dry'.

References

Académie nationale de pharmacie, 2006, 'A propos de l'automédication', rapport établi à la demande du Ministre de la santé et des solidarités, juin, 26 p. [www.acadpharm.org].

Aïach P. and Cèbe D., 1991, *Expression des symptômes et conduites de maladie*, Paris: Editions de l'Inserm/Doin.

Barthe J.F., 1990, 'Connaissance profane des symptômes et recours thérapeutiques', *Revue française de sociologie*, XXXI, 2: 283–296.

Baszanger I., 2010, 'Une autonomie incertaine : les malades et le système de soins', in: E. Hirsch (ed.), *Traité de bioéthique, II. Soigner la personne, évolutions, innovations thérapeutiques*, Toulouse: Erès, 189–198.

Blenkinsopp A. and Bradley C., 1996, 'Patients, society and the increase of self-medication', *BMJ*, 312: 629–632.

Bourdieu P., 1993, *La misère du monde*, Paris: Le Seuil, 1993.

Buclin T. and Ammon C. (eds), 2001, *L'automédication: pratique banale, motifs complexes*, Genève: Médecine et Hygiène, Cahiers Médico-Sociaux

CCNE, 2005, 'Refus de traitement et autonomie de la personne', *Les Cahiers du CCNE*, 44: 4–23.

Chauvel L., 2006, *Les classes moyennes à la dérive*, Paris : La République des idées/ Le Seuil.

Coulomb A., Baumelou A., 2007, 'Situation de l'automédication en France et perspectives d'évolution : marché, comportements, positions des acteurs', Rapport établi à la demande du ministère de la santé et de la protection sociale, 32 p.

CSA/CECOP, 2007, 'Les Français et l'automédication', enquête exclusive réalisée pour la Mutualité Française.

Dodier N., 2002, 'Recomposition de la médecine dans ses rapports avec la science. Les leçons du sida', *Santé publique et sciences sociales*, 8–9: 37–52.

Ehrenberg A., 2009, 'L'autonomie n'est pas un problème d'environnement, ou pourquoi il ne faut pas confondre interlocution et institution', in: M. Jouan and S. Laugier (eds), *Comment penser l'autonomie? Entre compétences et dépendances*, Paris: PUF (Éthique et philosophie morale), 219–235.

Eugeni E., 2011, 'Living a chronic illness: a condition between care and strategies', in: S. Fainzang and C. Haxaire (eds), *Of bodies and symptoms: anthropological perspectives on their social and medical treatment*, Tarragona: URV Publicacions, 111–126.

Faden R. and Beauchamp T.L., 1986, *A history and theory of informed consent*, New York: Oxford University Press.

Fainzang S., 2001b, *Médicaments et société. Le patient, le médecin et l'ordonnance*, Paris: Presses Universitaires de France.

Fainzang S., 2005, 'Religious attitudes toward prescriptions, medicines and doctors in France', *Culture, Medicine and Psychiatry*, 29, 4: 457–476.

Fainzang S., 2015, *An anthropology of lying: information in the doctor-patient relationship*, Farnham: Ashgate.

Gagnon E., 1995, 'Autonomie, normes de santé et individualité', in: J.F. Côté (ed.), *Individualismes et individualités*, Sillery, Montreal: Septentrion, 165–176.

Gillon R., 1985, 'Autonomy and the principle of respect for autonomy', *BMJ*, 290: 1806–1808.

Grand-Filaire A. (1992), 'Le bon usage du médicament en images', in: *Éducation pour la santé et bon usage du médicament*, Paris: Ed. du CFES.

Hamel J., 1998, 'Défense et illustration de la méthode des études de cas en sociologie et en anthropologie. Quelques notes et rappels: Figures de la connaissance', *Cahiers internationaux de sociologie*, 104: 121–138.

Hamel J., 2000, 'A propos de l'échantillon. De l'utilité de quelques mises au point', *Recherches qualitatives*, 21: 3–20.

Hoerni B., 1991, *L'autonomie en médecine. Nouvelles relations entre les personnes malades et les personnes soignantes*, Paris: Payot.

Jouan M. and Laugier S. (eds), 2009, *Comment penser l'autonomie? Entre compétences et dépendances*, Paris: Presses universitaires de France.

Kleinman A., 2002, 'Santé et stigmate', *Actes de la recherche en sciences sociales*, 3, 143: 97–99.

Laure P., 1998, 'Enquête sur les usagers de l'automédication: de la maladie à la performance', *Thérapie*, 53, 2: 127–135.

Lecomte T., 1999, 'Chiffres de l'automédication en France et à l'étranger', in: P. Queneau (ed), *Automédication, autoprescription, autoconsommation*. Paris: John Libbey, 49–56.

Lock M. and Nguyen V.K., 2010, *An anthropology of biomedicine*. Malden/Oxford: Wiley-Blackwell.

Massé R., 2003, *Ethique et santé publique. Enjeux, valeurs, normativités*, Québec: Presses de l'Université Laval.

Mauss M., 1966, *Sociologie et anthropologie*, Paris: Presses universitaires de France.

McLaughlin H., 2009, "What's in a Name: 'Client', 'Patient', 'Customer', 'Consumer', 'Expert by Experience', 'Service User'—What's Next?", *British Journal of Social Work*, 39: 1101–1117.

Molina N., 1988, *L'automédication*, Paris: PUF (Coll: Les champs de la santé).

Nichter M. and Vuckovic N., 1994, 'Agenda for an anthropology of pharmaceutical practice', *Social Science and Medicine*, 39, 11, 1509–1525.

Orfali K., 2003, 'L'émergence de l'éthique clinique: politique du sujet ou nouvelle catégorie clinique?', *Sciences sociales et santé*, 21, 2: 39–70.

Pierron J.-P., 2007, 'Une nouvelle figure du patient? Les transformations contemporaines de la relation de soins', *Sciences sociales et santé*, 25, 2: 43–66.

Rabeharisoa V. and Callon, M., 1999, *Le pouvoir des malades. L'Association française contre les myopathies et la Recherche*, Paris: Presses de l'Ecole des mines.

Raynaud D., 2008, 'Les déterminants du recours à l'automédication', *Revue Française des Affaires sociales*, 1: 81–94.

Rodriguez del Barrio L. (ed.), 2006, 'La gestion autonome de la médication en santé mentale. Bilan du suivi éducatif', projet pilote de collaboration entre les ressources alternatives et communautaires et le réseau public des services en santé mentale pour le renouvellement des pratiques, Erasme, Université de Montréal, 102 p.

Rogers A., 2010, 'Développer l'autogestion dans le cadre des maladies chroniques : l'exemple de l'expert patients programme (EPP)', in: I. Vincent, A. Loaec and C. Fournier (eds), *Modèles et pratiques en éducation du patient : apports internationaux*, 5è journées de la prévention, Paris, 2–3 avril 2009, Saint-Denis, INPES, collection Séminaires, 121–128.

Romeyer H., 2008, 'TIC et santé: entre information médicale et information de santé', *tic et société*, 2, 1 [http://ticetsociete.revues.org/365].

Rose N., 2005, 'In search of certainty: risk management in a biological age', *Journal of Public Mental Health*, 4, 3: 14–22.

Sand Andersen R., 2010, 'Anthropological perspectives on the biomedically defined problem of "patient delay"', in: S. Fainzang, H.E. Hem and M.B. Risor (eds), *The taste for knowledge: medical anthropology facing medical realities*, Copenhagen: Aarhus University Press, 57–68.

Schneewind J.B., 2001, *L'invention de l'autonomie. Une histoire de la philosophie morale moderne*, Paris: Gallimard.

Schneider C.E., 1998, *The practice of autonomy: patients, doctors, and medical decisions*, New York/Oxford: Oxford University Press.

Soum-Pouyalet F., 2007, 'Le patient acteur de la thérapie et l'évolution des normes professionnelles en cancérologie', in: F. Vedelago and M. Bouix (eds), 'Systèmes de santé et discours profanes', *Sociologie santé*, 2, 26: 123–134.

Thoër C., Pierret J. and Lévy J.J., 2008, 'Quelques réflexions sur des pratiques d'utilisation des médicaments hors cadre médical', *Drogues, santé et société*, 7, 1 : 19–54.

Tristram Engelhardt H. Jr., 2001, 'The many faces of autonomy', *Health Care Analysis*, 9, 283–297.

Van der Geest S., 2010, 'Patients as co-researchers? Views and experiences in Dutch medical anthropology', in: S. Fainzang, H.E. Hem and M.B. Risor (eds), *The taste for knowledge: medical anthropology facing medical realities*, Copenhagen: Aarhus University Press, 97–110.

Van der Geest S., Whyte S.R and Hardon A., 1996, 'The anthropology of pharmaceuticals: a biographical approach', *Annual Review of Anthropology*, 25: 153–178.

Vincent I., Loaec A and Fournier C. (eds), 2010, *Modèles et pratiques en éducation du patient: apports internationaux*, 5è journées de la prévention, Paris, 2–3 avril 2009, Saint-Denis, INPES, collection Séminaires.

Walger O., 2009, 'Empowerment et soutien social des personnes vivant avec un diabète: développement d'un outil d'évaluation à usage clinique', *Education du Patient et Enjeux de Santé*, 27, 1, 5–12.

Whyte S.R., Van der Geest S., Hardon H., 2002, *Social lives of medicines*, Cambridge: Cambridge University Press (college studies in medical anthropology).

Winance M., 2007, 'Dépendance versus autonomie … de la signification et de l'imprégnation de ces notions dans les pratiques médico-sociales', *Sciences sociales et santé*, 4: 83–91.

1 On the other side of the counter

To the joy of some and the sorrow of others, the French law of 30 June 2008 authorised open access to a certain number of medicines (Ministère de la santé, 2008). The question of open access engenders lively debates concerning access to non-prescription medicines on one hand, and direct access to medicines sold in pharmacies, not from behind the counter but in the users' space – also called, 'over the counter' – on the other. The debate becomes even more animated when the question of open access to drugs is coupled with that of their distribution, and when supermarkets attempt to challenge the monopoly of pharmacies on these products.

The stakes in the first part of the debate relate to the possibility that the subjects might do without a medical prescription for some medicines; those in the second part concern the possibility that the subjects might, under certain conditions, do without the mediation of a pharmacist and the third part deals with the potential for the subjects to do without their advice. In all of these cases, the different forms taken by this controversy centre on the question of the subjects' capacity to decide for themselves to acquire some types of medicines.

The economic dimension of this controversy is evident. It is indeed a deciding factor for some actors since self-medication generally involves the users paying for their own medicinal consumption. However, whether the actors are state legislators, the pharmaceutical industry, pharmacists, doctors or users, they all invoke a plethora of other reasons and arguments to make their cases. The link between the three parts, or levels of this debate (for or against self-medication, for or against open access to medicines and for or against medicinal sales in supermarkets), lies in the fact that one can contain the other without the opposite being necessarily the case. Thus, open access requires self-medication, but self-medication does not necessarily imply 'over the counter' access to medicines. Likewise, supermarket sales require open access which does not however necessarily imply that the drugs will be available in general stores. Thus the different levels of the controversy interlock to such a point that, in the debate at the second and third levels, the actors often mobilise arguments that endorse or denounce the object of the debate at a previous level.

The anthropologist's role when faced with this debate is not to take sides but to listen to the different voices being expressed and study the stakes and rationalities motivating them. It is thus not a case of joining the debate by adding another voice but of using a social science perspective to examine the discourses arising from this controversy. Here I will examine the positions and arguments of the different groups of actors concerned (public authorities, pharmaceutical industry, doctors, pharmacists and users) as they are expressed in the public sphere in order to grasp the cognitive, symbolic and ideological mechanisms so as to define the values that govern them and the logics that underpin them. To do this, I will mine resources from public statements, official websites, external communication documents and Internet discussion forums. Beyond the potential contradictions and ambiguities contained in these discourses, we will see, on one hand, that while they rely on some of the most popular values of our times, such as autonomy and responsibility, these values are sometimes invoked to defend opposing positions and, on the other hand, that the way they are used leads simultaneously to a limitation in their scope.[1]

The actors' positions

Public authorities

In order to reduce healthcare spending, the public authorities have adopted various measures to encourage the use of self-medication. Thus, they have taken a wide range of drugs off the list of medicines eligible for reimbursement and enacted a decree[2] promoting open access to 217 of them.[3] These measures are coupled with a discourse inviting patients to take responsibility for their ailments 'in benign situations'. Pursuant to this decree, which allows direct access to these medicines, pharmacists can now assign a space especially for over-the-counter drugs in their dispensary. This decision was made after the publication of a report on self-medication, called the Coulomb report, which recommended that the self-medication domain be organised by encouraging health professionals to support access to (i.e. 'accompany' the patient in his/her choice of) medicines in the pharmacy (Coulomb and Baumelou, 2007).

For the health ministry, the aim in facilitating direct access to medicines is primarily economic. The decision to remove eligibility for reimbursement from a series of medicines was intended to increase the proportion the users pay of their medicinal expenditure. With this new decree, the health minister said she wanted to make savings in health insurance costs and allow everyone to 'choose and compare' (La Mutualité Française, 2007). The idea of 'choice' is clear: the stated objective in allowing open access for certain pharmaceutical products is to promote competition in drug prices and, supposedly, to improve user buying power. In this way, the public authorities subscribe to the strategy of transferring state spending to the users in order to reduce public health insurance costs. But this measure comes with some precautions. It is not simply a case of 'offering competitive public prices and improving citizen buying power', but also of 'improving patient access to quality, appropriate information on the drugs they use without medical consultation', of 'offering them an informed choice accompanied with personalised advice', and of 'maintaining all the guarantees of accessibility, availability, and health safety provided by the pharmacies in France' (Health Ministry, 2008). The Coulomb report proposes that doctors play a part in these safety measures, that they should 'play a role of informing and advising' and 'also of verifying medicinal consumption, including outside of their own prescriptions'. Noting the information in the Coulomb report's chapter on international comparisons, the public authorities deplore that France is lagging behind in the domain of self-medication. Despite the growth in the self-medication market in the last few years (Blenkisopp and Bradley, 1996), the report notes that medicinal spending on self-medication products in France is low and relatively less than in other European countries (27 euros per person per year as opposed to 60 euros in Germany and 40 in the UK and Italy) (Le Pen, 2007).

Finally, as in the rhetoric of the Coulomb report, the public authorities perceive self-medication to be part of a 'responsible' economic policy on medicines and as one of the important elements in 'citizen responsibilisation'. The discourses expressed and the texts circulated in support of the decree in fact not only promote 'patient responsibility', but also their 'capacity'[4], and reiterate their intention of 'accompanying patients in their desire to be actors in their health' (Health Ministry, 2008). We will return to this point.

The pharmaceutical industry

The pharmaceutical industry, represented in particular by Afipa (Association Française de l'Industrie Pharmaceutique pour une Automédication responsable/ French Association of the Pharmaceutical Industry for Responsible Self-medication) and LEEM (Les Entreprises du Médicament/The pharmaceutical companies), supports the development of self-medication which it considers to be an 'important element of competitiveness for Europe and France' (Afipa, 2004). Bernard Lemoine, the vice-president delegate of LEEM, said: 'It is a fact today that most of the medicinal industry approves of the principle of self-medication, of family medication, meaning spontaneous drug purchases at the pharmacy' (La Mutualité Française, 2007). The industry is also largely in favour of open access to medicines. Afipa itself has long been lobbying for medicines to be available to consumers and placed on their side of the counter. But, like the public authorities, the industry defends the pharmacy monopoly on drug distribution[5] and recommends 'using a strong brand policy [...] to associate doctors with the promotion of self-medication' and to facilitate 'the oversight they can provide concerning the various medicines the patient is taking'.

Beyond the economic stakes of its position in the debate (Wallach, 2001), the industry tends to position itself in human, even political, terms by declaring that 'responsible' self-medication should be encouraged in order to 'meet the growing desire of individuals to take charge of their health' (Afipa, 2007). As Polillo and Mallet (2007) noted, 'the patient-consumer is both in opposition to and combined with the user-citizen, whose autonomy is asserted but who is simultaneously exploited in public policies and in professional, but above all, industrial strategies'.

For the industry, making patients 'responsible individuals' means making them choice-driven consumers, but it also means demonstrating a willingness to respond to patient demands. Thus the representative of *Bayer Santé familiale* declared: 'mind-sets are changing; [...] the French are convinced of the need to take care of their health capital in a responsible and more autonomous way' (Gautier, 2008), and Magalie Flachaire, the General Delegate of Afipa, said 'we are starting from the observation that our co-citizens are capable of identifying small health problems and taking them in hand....' (Afipa, 2007). The industry therefore asserts both patient rights and patient competence.

The doctors

According to an Afipa-Institut Louis Harris inquiry in 2004, 57 per cent of doctors are supportive of self-medication. They think that 'excessive time' is dedicated to 'small complaints' within their practices, and that this 'precious time' could be given over to prevention and caring for more serious pathologies (Afipa, 2004). We can easily imagine indeed that some doctors support self-medication in that it would empty their waiting rooms somewhat and allow them to respond more rapidly to the consultation needs of patients with serious pathologies. This is a powerful argument in the context of a deficit in the medical demography where self-medication could be a means of mitigating the shortage of doctors. This position is defended by the economist Claude Le Pen, for whom self-medication is a solution to the declining medical demography which makes accessing a doctor more difficult (Le Pen, 2003).

However, many doctors express strong reservations regarding self-medication. The French Medical Association bulletin echoed this feeling by saying that while it has 'some advantages', it also carries 'numerous adverse effects' (Pouillard, 2001). While self-medication 'can be tolerated when it extends an already established therapy' and can be 'useful to temporarily attenuate a troublesome condition with a short-term medication, while waiting for a medical opinion, [...] it can become very dangerous if it is used for an extended period, if a medical consultation is not sought or if it is used imprudently' (Pouillard, 2001). Thus, self-medication is often considered to be a 'risky practice', risks resulting from 'prescriptions without specific therapeutic justification' or 'non-controlled practices of self-medication that do not follow the rules of use: no verification of posology, treatment duration, medicinal interactions, iatrogenic or allergic reactions or medicinal expiry dates (family pharmacy cabinets)'. Michel Chassang, the president of the Confederation of French Medical Syndicates, believes that the development of self-medication leads a symptom to be associated with a medicine, an association which is detrimental to appropriate healthcare for the patient. As such, he thinks it is both dangerous and can foster illusions. He is worried about 'the evolution of our society where bypassing the doctor has become a national sport'

(La Mutualité Française, 2007). Moreover, many doctors fear the potential for diagnostic delay inherent in self-medication, since patients are not capable, they believe, of knowing the difference between a benign symptom and a serious one. And so, they think patients should turn to their expertise since their knowledge is indispensable to appropriate healthcare provision, for all pathologies.[6] In these conditions, open access is even more disapproved of by the majority of doctors. Yet, subjects are partly socialised and coached in self-medication by some doctors themselves. In this regard, the medical body is not homogenous.[7] The majority however consider that despite 'the dangers linked to consumer ignorance', the medical world 'should today take the practice of self-medication into account', and that it 'should be guided by precise advice to ill people' (Queneau *et al.*, 2004), in consideration of their 'demand for autonomy'.

Pharmacists

In a debate initiated on the Internet by the *60 millions de consommateurs* magazine concerning open access to medicines,[8] in which numerous pharmacists took part, an assortment of opinions can be found. Some were outright hostile to self-medication itself, others to open access to medicines, or to drug sales in supermarkets, covering all three parts of the controversy. Some were in line with the industry, others took the doctors' side, while a third group took intermediary positions – being in favour of self-medication for example but against open access. On the other hand, as can be expected, they all condemned supermarket sales, though for very different reasons. The positions against self-medication itself are most often justified by evoking the danger it represents: 'It is in the USA that there are the most hospitalisations resulting from self-medication. No medicine is harmless! They are all dangerous!' one pharmacist said (60 millions, 2008). Others accept the idea of self-medication but not open access, even for cases said to be 'benign'. One pharmacist wrote: 'self-service sales of harmful molecules are inadmissible', and used as an example the fact that 'taking aspirin when pregnant can seriously harm the fœtus'. Another web user pointed out that 'a sore throat and a headache can be the first signs of scarlet fever', and that 'to avoid complications, a correct treatment must be administered as soon as the symptoms appear, symptoms that require serious investigation'. This is indeed the point of view of the National Academy of Pharmacy (2006) who stated that open access is 'an imprudence detrimental to public health, considering the long-standing habits of our country', and who, on this basis, is against leaving drugs of any sort in open access, even within a pharmacy.

While some pharmacists approve of self-medication, they nevertheless all stress, loud and clear, the importance of their role in advising consumers which potentially implies that the medicines should be kept behind the counter. Their hostility to open access is sometimes linked to the risk that it could boost consumption (Légaré, 2008). Thus, for F. Abecassis, the spokesperson for the *Pharmaciens en colère* collective (*'Angry Pharmacists'*), medicines are not everyday consumption goods (60 millions, 2008). 'If medicines are made available over the counter in order to consume them at a lower cost, French people will consume them even more when they are already consuming too many' (60 millions, 2008). In the same vein, the Order of Pharmacists says that 'medicines should not be confused with merchandise'. Still others believe that open access is not unreasonable as long as they can 'accompany' the patient, meaning retaining their exclusive right to distribute medicines.

All in all, several different logics underpin the points of view expressed by the pharmacists (Logan, 1983). Thus we find: defence of the corporation or the profession; defence of consumers (with a denunciation of the appetites of the supermarkets or pharmaceutical laboratories); and defence of public health. These different logics are sometimes combined. Defence of public health, defence of the profession and defence of the consumers all merge on the theme of the risks posed by self-medication, caused by what is thought of as user incompetence (Fainzang, 2001a): 'Users do not know how to recognise symptoms and cannot know if they are banal or not'; 'Most French people do not know the difference between aspirin and paracetamol'. Noting this paucity of medical information leads some pharmacists to deem the situation irremediable ('It is irresponsible on the part of the state; we know very well that people will never read the counter-indications and an accident can happen so quickly') and to lament the incapability of users to correctly self-medicate despite the information they might receive ('It is an illusion to think that people will responsibly self-medicate; how can we be sure that the users will take the correct dose, for the correct amount of time, if no-one is guiding them?'; 'France is not ready for self-medication'). Despite the recommendations of those who believe in user education (Balcou-Debussche, 2006),[9] some pharmacists seem to believe people are uneducable, even for benign cases. In this regard, while paternalism is often evoked to describe the doctor–patient relationship (Prayle and Brazier, 1998; Charles, Gafni and Whelan, 1999; Freidson, 2004; Rameix, 1997; Fainzang, 2015; Bergeron, 2007), we can note that it also partly characterises the pharmacist–user relationship The patient is no longer this 'capable' individual recognised by the industry and the public authorities, but one who requires professional expertise at all times.

The users

While the majority of users[10] are in favour of self-medication, opinions are more circumspect about open access, either for therapeutic or economic reasons. Some warmly welcome this measure, while hoping to see the pharmacists retain their advisory role and that the supermarkets are not allowed to take over the sector: 'Is there not a risk in buying these substances at the same time as eggs or chocolate? The oversight carried out by pharmacists during the sale is not just a myth, it prevents numerous medicinal accidents,' one web user declared. Others however worry about the consequences of open access precisely because it may herald an opening for supermarket sales which would lead to a trivialisation of medicines: 'Medicines are not sweets as represented by *Leclerc* (a French supermarket chain) in their advert with this necklace that looks like the sweet necklaces we used to eat when we were children!' This argument is however challenged by those who note that pharmacies also sell sweets. In contrast, a certain number of users have a positive view of the potential consequences of such access in supermarkets. A CSA/Cecop study in February 2007 indeed showed that 24 per cent of respondents said they would willingly buy medicines elsewhere than in pharmacies, and this figure rose to 34 per cent amongst those who regularly practiced self-medication (CSA/CECOP, 2007).

On a strictly economic level, the decree also provokes contrasting reactions: some deplore the potential effects of a drop in prices and fear this measure will incite people to consume more, while others appreciate the fact that the decree obliges pharmacists to display the drug prices, and still others think, to the contrary, that it will cause drug prices to rise. The debate is muddied by uncertainties on the effects open access will have on prices. Indeed, it is also for economic reasons that some people perceive the possibility of supermarket medicinal sales in a positive light. In this context, the argument regarding the advisory role of pharmacists is challenged by those who imply that, in any case, this 'advisory' role is a myth: 'When you go into a pharmacy, they don't ask you anything more than in a supermarket; you are served and that is it. Pharmacists have become shopkeepers; they are there to make sales and profits, that's all!'

Finally, the availability of over-the-counter drugs, in both pharmacies and supermarkets, is warmly welcomed by certain users who appreciate being able to choose for themselves and resented being infantilised when they did not have direct access to these medicines, as shown by these statements: 'We are capable of taking care of our little problems!' or 'We are not kids; we do actually know what we are doing!' They affirm their desire to take their health into their own hands on the grounds that they possess sufficient competence.

As we have seen, this controversy is developing around various different issues, such as danger for example, which some associate with open access to medicines, and others simply with self-medication in itself. However, beyond the stakes governing these issues, the presuppositions they are based on and the contradictions they contain, it is appropriate to question the way in which certain aspects of the debate are organised in its dialogic and rhetorical dimensions.

Discussion points

A further examination of the arguments developed by the actors to defend their positions requires some additional comments which lead us to an analysis of the social treatment of the notion of autonomy.

Information and advertising

Everyone agrees that patient education is essential in self-medication, but they do not all concur on what this education should contain. Both Christian Saout, the vice-president of the *Collectif Inter-Associatif sur la Santé* that federates the different patient associations, and Jean-Pierre Davant, the president of the *Mutualité Francaise*, believe that one step for successful self-medication is 'better information for patients'. The latter thinks patients should be encouraged to always read the accompanying leaflet and verify the INN (international non-proprietary name) to make sure they do not take the same product twice under two different brand names so as to prevent excessive doses (La Mutualité Française, 2007). This position is in opposition to that of the industry which calls for the promotion of brands, thus blurring the boundaries between information and advertising. Indeed advertising is an important stake here since it is authorised for medicines classified as 'self-medication'. Representatives of the industry justify it by a desire to see the patients 'better informed' and to provide them with the same type of choice as for any object of consumption. On this point we should note the contradiction in their discourse since they also affirm the need for a pharmaceutical monopoly based on the fact that 'self-medication' drugs are potentially dangerous products just like drugs available under medical prescription only, which suggests that these are *not consumption products like any other*, but they ask nevertheless to be able to advertise these self-medication drugs *as they do for other consumption goods*. In truth, information and advertising cannot be assimilated, any more than a means of information can be confused with a means of promotion. However, the French National Academy of Pharmacy (2006) appears to make this confusion in recommending that the pharmaceutical industry provide improved information to patients to enable medicinal use without medical prescription. As the *Revue Prescrire* reiterates: 'True patient autonomy requires the provision of trustworthy and independent information on diseases and the therapeutic, and above all medicinal, options' (*Revue Prescrire*, 2008).

Between doctors and pharmacists: a conflict of competencies

Examining the actors' positions raises the question of the respective roles of doctors and pharmacists (Aïach, Fassin and Saliba, 1994; Saliba, 1994). The ideas of *accompaniment* and *advice* developed by the public authorities and the industry in reference to the pharmacists' role imply that they should be able to question the patients about their affliction to 'guide them in their choices'. What should be understood by that? That the pharmacist should take on the doctor's role? In everyday language as well as legally, a doctor's knowledge results in prescriptions, while the pharmacist's knowledge is used to provide 'advice'. Should the pharmacist's 'advice' substitute the doctor's 'prescription', the only difference between them being that the 'advised' products are not reimbursable? The French National Academy of Pharmacy (2006) appears to believe this since, in a statement regarding the responsibilities of pharmacists, it affirms their role as 'prescribing pharmacists, major actors in public health'. In these conditions, what is the meaning of the pharmacist's 'guidance' or 'advice' concerning users' decisions, if it is not to place them in a position of a prescriber and a salesperson at the same time, entailing a collusion between therapeutic and commercial interests?

In turn, the role of 'advisory doctor' also raises a difficulty. To be more precise, the place assigned to doctors in the context of self-medication reveals a contradiction. Since, if they are expected to '*guide* patient self-medication' or 'verify medicinal consumption, including outside of their own prescriptions', it is hard to see how this role is different from the one they play during their usual activity of consulting and prescribing, nor what this role of 'informing and advising' means, if it is not simply the obligation for the user to pay for the treatment, justified by replacing the term 'prescription' with that of 'advice', just as is happening for pharmacists. The contents of the terms 'prescribe' and 'advise' become vague and uncertain. Has the doctors' role come to compete with that of the pharmacists? And in what way is this self-medication? Does being told (or being 'advised' or 'prescribed') what one should take still count as self-medication? And subsequently where does the personal nature of the choice to self-medicate reside?

The spectre of the family medicine cabinet

The notion of 'self-medication drugs', widely used by the public authorities, the industry and pharmacists alike to designate medicines with optional medical prescription, introduces confusion. Strictly speaking, 'self-medication drugs' cannot be confused with the drugs *taken as self-medication*. In this regard, the 'prescription of self-medication drugs' that the Afipa would like to see developed appears an aporia. If we want to take into account the reality of self-medication practices, and free ourselves from any normative posture, we must admit that the patients willingly rely on their family medicine cabinet and that self-medication cannot be reduced to simply buying medicines since it can also involve taking medicines already in one's possession.[11] This practice attracts widespread disapproval. For J.-P. Davant, President of the French Mutuality, self-medication should not be 'behaviour consisting of rummaging through the medical cabinet to use the remains of medicines previously prescribed by a GP for similar symptoms [but] a response consisting of going to the pharmacy to find a treatment for a benign and easily-resolved affliction' (La Mutualité Française, 2007). Equally, Afipa thinks that responsible self-medication should not be confused with 'the irrational use of former prescriptions'. For his part, Gilles Bonnefond of the French Syndicate of Dispensary Pharmacists declared: 'We distinguish between self-medication and the medicine cabinet. We all have an interest today in working together to empty these medicine cabinets. Because these tail-ends of treatments, these remnants, are potentially extremely dangerous and increase the risk of iatrogenic results' (La Mutualité Française, 2007). This view echoes that of the French National Academy of Pharmacy (2006) that self-medication taken in the sense of 'individual behaviour consisting of treating oneself' relying on 'products stored at home, constitutes an error that can harm patient health'. The act of self-medicating appears therefore to necessarily require a purchase since the use of previously bought medicines is not condoned. It excludes 'the "notorious" medicine cabinet' that poses the problem of 'misuse', in the words of the Coulomb report (Coulomb and Baumelou, 2007: 1).

However, taking recourse to the pharmacy cabinet should not be considered, a priori, as misuse. Indeed, if the symptom is familiar, why should the user not 'rummage in his/her pharmacy cabinet'? Why should this cabinet be 'excluded', or even 'emptied'? Is it so that the pharmacist can sell the patient the same medicinal product a second time, if it turns outs that the pharmacist advises exactly the same drug as the patient already possesses? The argument that the decree enabling open access to medicines is economically beneficial for patients whose buying power is in jeopardy (Petryna, Lakoff and Kleinman, 2006) does not stand up to scrutiny. If the aim is to prevent the patient from taking an out-of-date medicine, the patient education that everyone recommends appears thus not to include teaching citizens to look at the expiry date on the boxes in their possession, which eviscerates the discourse on the need to inform the patient.

Autonomous self-medication?

The different actors' arguments are peppered with thoughts on the competence of ill people, as we have seen. Recommending self-medication, and *a fortiori* open access, relies on the notions of patient 'responsibility', 'autonomy' and their 'ability to handle their health', with the stated concern of answering to the very wishes of individuals. It is the idea of helping the patients out, of *responsibilising* them, and giving them the possibility of being *enlightened actors* in their health-care that should be guiding the development of self-medication. The controversy thus touches on political considerations concerning the individual, in his/her role as a competent, adult citizen. Self-medication and open access are in fact particularly appreciated by the users themselves who would sometimes rather not pass through the mediation of professionals (that of doctors or even that of pharmacists), and see in them a means of emancipation from this authority.[12] The industry itself, beyond the need for product sales – that self-medication and open access prove very opportunely to increase – declares that self-medication 'is a cultural and social reality in the sense that people are undertaking more and more of the management of their own health' and that 'the development of self-medication corresponds with a profound evolution in mind-sets and attitudes towards health' (Afipa, 2004).[13] Equally, the public authorities, beyond their aim to reduce health insurance costs, state that self-medication is necessary to allow ill people to take charge of their health in conformity with 'their desire to be actors of their health', and thus to 'respond to their expectations' (Health Ministry, 2008).[14]

A fundamental element of the industry rhetoric as well as that of public authorities is the need to show how seriously the values newly expressed by the users and heralded by the patient associations are taken. In support of a decree where the stakes are clearly economic, the various actors produce discourses asserting and advocating the possibility for users to exercise what is presented as a competence and a right. It is as if using the argument of responsibility/responsibilisation and autonomy/autonomisation (in all its different variants) is necessary in all rhetoric in order to achieve the aims, be they exclusively economic. Conversely, the actors opposed to open access, or even self-medication, refute this user competence. To say that users are 'not able' and 'not ready' to self-medicate, that they don't know the difference between medicines, that they will never read the accompanying leaflet, or to consider them uneducable, is to deny their status as competent adults. But it is also paradoxically with reference to the characterisation of the 'new patient' (not being passive, willing to be informed, etc.) that they are sometimes refused this ability to self-medicate: the view of the French National Academy of Pharmacy (2006) is that 'today's patients have changed; they want more information, more explanations but not to be abandoned in front of a mute display case loaded with medicines'. It is therefore in response to modern-day patient aspirations that the Academy refuses the idea of open access. The concept of the contemporary patient, endowed with these new qualities, is thus invoked to defend opposing positions.

However, while affirming this autonomy, its defenders do set some limits, as shown by the injunctions to not take recourse to the medicine cabinet. These limits can be identified in the therapeutic reasons they evoke which imply that taking a medicine from the medicine cabinet necessarily shows bad usage and involves taking a risk. This effectively amounts to considering individuals as unable and uneducable and, ultimately, as non-autonomous and irresponsible.

The affirmation of autonomy has always been closely linked to the recognition of competence or, in more technical terms, capacity (Beauchamp and Childress, 1979; Gillon, 1985; Gagnon, 1995, 1998; Hoerni, 1991; Schneider, 1998; Mackenzie and Stoljar, 2000; Schneewind, 2001; Meyers, 2004; Jouan and Laugier, 2009; Baszanger, 2010). We cannot imagine recognising a person's autonomy if he/she is deprived of the means to exercise it. Autonomy requires the subject to have a faculty of discernment (Gillon, 1985) since an autonomous person is, in the CCNE's (2005) words, capable of 'understanding medical information and undertaking critical reflection on the subject' and of 'reflecting on personal objectives and deciding independently to act in conformity with that reflection' (p. 23), echoing the Kantian view that autonomy is the capacity to make use of ones' own reason.

In fact, there is no certainty as to whether the user is genuinely recognised as autonomous in the field of self-medication, even if he/she is granted open access to medicines. Through the discourses arising from the current debate on self-medication, we can note that the injunction not to use the family medicine cabinet and to always go to a pharmacy to buy medicine – from one side of the counter or the other – makes subject autonomy a beguiling illusion.

Analysing the arguments used and values assigned by the actors regarding self-medication and open access reveals that the controversy, based on a battle of interests that differ for each group of actors, is inseparable from a war of words: 'oversight', 'control', 'prescription', 'advice', 'accompaniment' etc., each word referring to different realities, rights and statuses. But, whether it is for therapeutic or economic reasons, or whether one is arguing to defend corporate prerogatives or to protect patients from the danger they expose themselves to, it is the language of autonomy that provides weight and legitimacy to the discourses. We could see here the fact that responsibility and autonomy, satellite notions of the affirmation of the individual, are widely advocated in our times, under the growing influence of the Anglo-Saxon model. But there is more. It all takes place as if the various actors cannot simply promote the economic reasons, and that they have to find other justifications and arguments likely to provide their positions with legitimacy and dignity. Public authorities, the industry, doctors, pharmacists and users alike integrate these notions into their discourses, although from differing perspectives, since it is in the name of these values that open access is approved by some and condemned by others. In the public authorities' discourse, the decree concerning open access to medicines, which could potentially prove unpopular since it involves higher spending for the users and a redistribution of power to the detriment of doctors (even sometimes pharmacists), needed an ideological dressing to make it acceptable. Making the patient a 'responsible' agent, 'an actor in health' and 'autonomous' in order to make him/her a consumer who pays for his/her expenses, functions as a sort of rhetorical device, a magic spell that renders the discourse acceptable. As the cornerstone of an apparent consensus, autonomy has become an incantation. The users are no longer the only ones demanding a role as actors; this demand is now being made with other voices (the public authorities, the industry and some pharmacists), other stakeholders in the controversy, who want to see the users playing this role as inseparable from that of an autonomous consumer. In some ways, by invoking the values of responsibility and autonomy, these diverse groups of actors drive and support their promotion despite themselves.

However, the rhetoric of the discourse is based on handling, if not manipulating, these notions. While the users demand autonomy in order to be able to be actors in their health, authors of their actions and freely responsible for their decisions, its use by the public authorities, the industry and to a certain extent health professionals aims to render them consumers who pay for their own health spending but are not, for all that, capable of making the right decision. A responsible patient appears to be reduced to simply being a patient accountable for his/her choices to consume. It is interesting to note in this regard that the French word 'responsabilité' encompasses both responsibility and accountability, the specific meaning depending on the context in which it is used. The discourse in French can thus easily conflate the two. On this point, Hunter (2010), following Tristram Engelhardt (2001), observed that 'accountability has always been the flip side of the autonomous coin in moral philosophy' (p. 1547). As such, this loudly demanded autonomy takes a different meaning: far from being the political proclamation of individual capacity for self-determination in line with freely chosen rules without submitting to an authority, we in fact end up with a disdainful claim of individuals' incapacity to manage their family pharmacy and of the necessity to teach them how to buy new drugs, at their own cost, under the advice of pharmacists, or even doctors. The statements concerning individual 'responsibility' and 'autonomy' have paradoxical and fatal consequences: as they plead for the promotion of these values, they slowly empty them of all their substance.

Notes

1 My interest in this dispute is not intended to situate this analysis in a sociology of controversy or public debates (Callon *et al.*, 2001; Chateauraynaud, 2002; Urfalino, 2007) but to examine, based on this debate, the social treatment of the notion of 'autonomy' applied to the user in the domain of self-medication.
2 Cf. Decree no. 2008–641 of 30 June 2008.
3 A number that has since risen. According to Giroud (2011), this figure had risen to 390 in 2010.
4 'Patients have changed a lot in the last few years: they are better informed, and better able to decide to take charge of their benign pathologies without systematically resorting to a doctor' (Health Ministry, 2008).
5 It should be noted however that the industry is not in favour of removing eligibility for reimbursement from drugs, in that this leads to a decrease in sales volumes because of the meaning the removal of reimbursement takes in the eyes of users, who tend to assimilate this with insufficient efficacy (Afipa, 2004).
6 This hostility to self-medication is not new. It is in fact anchored in the discourse of doctors to such a point that, for a long time, their disapproval led patients to dissimulate the practice (cf. Fainzang, 2001b).
7 The doctors that Anne Véga puts in the category of 'little prescribers' thus educate their patients to wait for further developments and take on the responsibility themselves (Vega, 2011: 183).
8 Here it is not a case of a discussion list as studied by Akrich and Méadel (2002) for example, but of a forum created by *60 millions de consommateurs* on their website, where web users are invited to express their opinions for or against open access to medicines.
9 Jean Parrot, President of the National Order of Pharmacists, stressed the need for patient education (La Mutualité Française, 2007).
10 Despite the widespread use of the term 'patient' in most of the discourses and texts relating to self-medication, it would be preferable to say 'user' to refer to the subjects' position as consumers.
11 According to a study carried out by the CSA-TMO institute on behalf of the DGS [General Directorate of Health] in 2002 (DGS/CSA-TMO santé, 2002), the very first resort when faced with a pain or a symptom is to look in the family medicine cabinet. A majority of people reuse previously prescribed medicines kept in home when the person to be treated is an adult.
12 See the study carried out by the Institut CSA/Cecop for the French Mutuality (Mutualité Française), where 55 per cent of respondents associated self-medication with autonomous health management *without recourse to intermediaries* (Press release of the French Mutuality/Communiqué de presse de la Mutualité Française – 21/03/2007).
13 As a matter of fact, this phenomenon is not specific to France (see *Consumerism in Health Care*, AETNA, www.aetna.com/aboutlaoti/aetna_perspective/consumerism_healthcare.html, cited by Hunter, 2010).
14 The public authorities' discourse, primarily motivated by the desire to reduce health costs – a concern echoed by Rothman (2001) and Hunter (2010) in their observations on medical consumerism in the United States – draws heavily on the rhetoric of autonomy to promote self-medication.

References

60 millions de consommateurs, 2009, 'La vente des médicaments en libre accès dans les pharmacies?' [www.60millions-mag.com].

Afipa, 2004, *Livre blanc: contribution de l'Afipa à la réflexion sur l'automédication*, Afipa document, Paris, 81 p.

Afipa, 2007, 'Pour une automédication responsable: le libre accès aux médicaments sans ordonnance en pharmacie. 1ère étape du parcours de soins du patient', document, 27 p. [www.afipa.org/afipa/pdf/4178_afipa_communique_presse_24_oct_2007.pdf].

Aïach P., Fassin D. and Saliba, J., 1994, 'Crise, pouvoir et légitimité', in P. Aïach and D. Fassin (eds), *Les métiers de la santé, enjeux de pouvoir et quête de légitimité*, Paris: Anthropos-Economica, 9–42.

Akrich M. and Méadel C., 2002, 'Prendre ses médicaments / prendre la parole: les usages des médicaments par les patients dans les listes de discussion électroniques', *Sciences Sociales et Santé*, 20, 1 (special issue: 'Les médicaments : des prescriptions aux usages'): 89–116.

Balcou-Debussche M., 2006, *L'éducation des malades chroniques. Une approche ethno-sociologique*, Paris: Editions des archives contemporaines.

Baszanger I., 2010, 'Une autonomie incertaine: les malades et le système de soins', in: E. Hirsch (ed.), *Traité de bioéthique, II. Soigner la personne, évolutions, innovations thérapeutiques*, Toulouse: Erès, 189–198.

Beauchamp T. and Childress, J., 1979, *Principles of biomedical ethics*, New York: Oxford University Press.

Bergeron H., 2007, 'Les transformations du 'colloque singulier' médecin/patient: quelques perspectives sociologiques', Colloque Chaire Santé de Sciences Po / Collectif interas-sociatif sur la Santé sur: *Les droits des malades et des usagers du système de santé, une législature plus tard*, 10 p. [www.cso.edu/upload/pdf_actualites/bergeron-colloque-mars2007.pdf].

Blenkinsopp A. and Bradley C., 1996, 'Patients, society and the increase of self-medication', *BMJ*, 312: 629–632.

Bond C.M. and Bradley C., 1996, 'Over the counter drugs: the interface between the community pharmacist and patients', *BMJ*, 312: 758–760.

Callon M., Lascoumes P. and Barthe Y., 2001, *Agir dans un monde incertain. Essai sur la démocratie technique*, Paris: Le Seuil.

CCNE, 2005, 'Refus de traitement et autonomie de la personne', *Les Cahiers du CCNE*, 44: 4–23.

Charles C., Gafni A. and Whelan T., 1999, 'Decision-making in the physician-patient Encounter: revisiting the shared treatment decision-making model'. *Social Science & Medicine*, 49: 651–661.

Chateauraynaud F., 2002, 'Prospero, Une Méthode d'Analyse des Controverses Publiques', in: P. Blanchard and T. Ribémont (eds), *Méthodes et outils des sciences sociales – Innovation et renouvellement, Cahiers Politiques*, Paris: L'Harmattan, 61–84.

Coulomb A. and Baumelou A., 2007, 'Situation de l'automédication en France et perspectives d'évolution: marché, comportements, positions des acteurs', Rapport établi à la demande du ministère de la santé et de la protection sociale, 32 p.

CSA/CECOP, 2007, 'Les Français et l'automédication', enquête exclusive réalisée pour la Mutualité Française.

Deschandol P., 1998, 'Le droit des patients: le patient entre citoyen et usager', *Décision santé*, 135: 15–23.

DGS/CSA-TMO santé, 2002, *Enquête sur l'automédication*, October.

Fainzang S., 2001a, 'Cohérence, raison et paradoxe. L'anthropologie de la maladie aux prises avec la question de la rationalité', *Ethnologies comparées,* 3 [http://recherche.univ-montp3.fr/cerce/r3/s.f.htm].

Fainzang S., 2001b, *Médicaments et société. Le patient, le médecin et l'ordonnance*, Paris: Presses Universitaires de France.

Fainzang S., 2015, *An anthropology of lying: information in the doctor-patient relationship*, Farnham: Ashgate.

Friedson E., 1984, *La profession médicale*. Paris: Payot ('Médecine et sociétés').

Gagnon E., 1995, 'Autonomie, normes de santé et individualité', in J.F. Côté (ed.), *Individualismes et individualités*, Sillery, Montreal: Septentrion, 165–176.

Gagnon E., 1998, 'L'avènement médical du sujet. Les avatars de l'autonomie en santé', *Sciences sociales et santé*, 16, 1: 49–74.

Gautier C., 2008, 'Vers plus d'autonomie pour le patient', *Le Monde* (*Les cahiers de la compétitivité*, spécial Santé), 18 June, p. v.

Gillon R., 1985, 'Autonomy and the principle of respect for autonomy', *BMJ*, 290: 1806–1808.

Giroud J.-P., 2011, *Médicaments sans ordonnance, les bons et les mauvais*, Paris: Ed. de la Martinière.

Health Ministry (Ministère de la santé), 2008, 'Libre accès de certains médicaments devant le comptoir', Dossier Presse, 1 July [www.sante-jeunesse-sports.gouv.fr/actualite-presse/presse-sante].

Hoerni B., 1991, *L'autonomie en médecine. Nouvelles relations entre les personnes malades et les personnes soignantes*, Paris: Payot.

Hunter, N.D., 2010, 'Rights talk and patient subjectivity: the role of autonomy, equality and participation norms'. *Georgetown Law Faculty Publications and Other Works*. Paper 473. [http://scholarship.law.georgetown.edu/facpub/473].

Jouan M. and Laugier S. (eds), 2009, *Comment penser l'autonomie? Entre compétences et dépendances*, Paris: Presses universitaires de France.

La Mutualité Française, 2007, 'L'Automédication: recul ou progrès?', Actes du colloque: 'Regard croisés sur l'automédication. Un colloque de la FNMF', Paris, 21 March 2007.

Le Pen C., 2003, *Automédication et Santé Publique: le 'Service médical rendu' par les médicaments d'automédication*, CLP-Santé Paris, report made in collaboration with l'AFIPA.

Le Pen C., 2007, 'La consommation médicamenteuse dans 5 pays européens: une réévaluation', Paris: LEEM.

Légaré N., 2008, 'Les médicaments en vente libre comme substances d'abus: revue d'un phénomène méconnu', *Drogues, santé et société*, 7, 1: 129–151.

Logan K., 1983, 'The role of pharmacists and over the counter medications in the health care system of a Mexican city', *Medical Anthropology*, VII, 3: 68–89.

Mackenzie C. and Stoljar N. (eds), 2000, *Relational autonomy: feminist perspectives on autonomy, agency, and the social self*, New York/Oxford: Oxford University Press.

Meyers C., 2004, 'Cruel choices: autonomy and critical care decision-making', *Bioethics*, 18, 2: 104–119.

Ministère de la santé, 2008, 'Libre accès de certains médicaments devant le comptoir', Dossier Presse, 1 July [www.sante-jeunesse-sports.gouv.fr/actualite-presse/presse-sante].

National Academy of Pharmacy (Académie nationale de pharmacie), 2006, 'A propos de l'automédication', rapport établi à la demande du Ministre de la santé et des solidarités, June, 26 p. [www.acadpharm.org].

Petryna A., Lakoff A. and Kleinman A. (eds), 2006, *global pharmaceuticals: ethics, markets, practices*, Durham: Duke University Press.

Polillo R. and Mallet J.-O., 2007, 'Face aux professions et au management, les patients dans la redistribution des pouvoirs: éléments de comparaison en France et en Italie', in: F. Vedelago and M. Bouix (eds), 'Systèmes de santé and discours profanes', *Sociologie santé*, 2, 26: 175–185.

Pouillard J., 2001, 'Risques et limites de l'automédication', *Bulletin de l'Ordre des Médecins*, April [http://bulletin.conseil-national.medecin.fr/Archives].

Prayle D. and Brazier M., 1998, 'Supply of medicines: paternalism, autonomy and reality', *Journal of Medical Ethics*, 24, 2: 93–98.

Queneau P., Froudarakis M., Salvador M, Villani P. and Vital-Durand D., 2004, 'Automédication concernant les antalgiques', *in* : P. Queneau and G. Ostermann (eds), *Le médecin, le malade et la douleur*. Paris: Masson, 389–398.

Rameix S., 1997, 'Du paternalisme des soignants à l'autonomie des patients', *Laennec*, 10, 1: 10–15.

Rothman D.J., 2001, 'The origins and consequences of patient autonomy: a 25-year retrospective', *Health Care Analysis*, 9, 3: 255–264.

Saliba J., 1994, 'Les paradigmes des professions de santé', in: P. Aïach and D. Fassin (eds), *Les métiers de la santé. Enjeux de pouvoir et quête de légitimité*, Paris: Anthropos, 43–85.

Schneewind J.B., 2001, *L'invention de l'autonomie. Une histoire de la philosophie morale moderne*, Paris: Gallimard.

Schneider C.E., 1998, *The practice of autonomy: patients, doctors, and medical decisions*, New York/Oxford: Oxford University Press.

Tristram Engelhardt H. Jr., 2001, 'The many faces of autonomy', *Health Care Analysis*, 9: 283–297.

Urfalino P., 2007, 'Médicaments et société. Enjeux contemporains. Introduction', *Annales*, 62è année, 2: 269–272.

Vega A., 2011, 'Le partage des responsabilités en médecine. Une approche socio-anthropologique des pratiques soignantes', report for the CNAMTS, 199 p.

Wallach I., 2001, '"Automédication responsible": un partenariat pharmaciens-industriels pour le bienfait des consommateurs', in: T. Buclin and C. Ammon (eds), *L'automédication, pratique banale, motifs complexes*, Genève: Editions Médecine et Hygiène, 167–171.

2 Self-medication, between signs and symptoms

The identification of symptoms is a decisive element in the therapeutic itinerary of individuals in that it leads to a specific course of action. There exists abundant literature on the subject. These studies investigated the meaning of symptoms in diverse societies and the role they play in the process of deciding to seek medical care (Kleinman, 1980; Good and Good, 1981).

Symptoms and therapeutic strategies

A large number of anthropological works have looked into the place occupied by symptoms in various cognitive systems. Young's (1976) work is a prime example. He demonstrated that the perception of symptoms is a collective phenomenon. He wrote: 'If we want to learn the social meaning of sickness, we must understand that "signs", whatever their genesis, become symptoms because they are expressed, elicited, and perceived in socially acquired ways' (1976: 14). More generally, anthropologists have endeavoured to show that the meaning assigned to symptoms is the result of a cultural construction, and that each society has its own way of conceiving illness and its signs, whether in the fields of mental or somatic health (Delvecchio-Good *et al.* 1994; Martinez-Hernaez, 2000; Hay, 2008). Martinez-Hernaez, for example, examined, based on contemporary psychiatric data in particular, the question of whether symptoms are physical signs of an illness or forms of symbolic and cultural expression, and what they signify. He showed that, whilst they are psychological or physio-pathological, symptoms are very much cultural manifestations. This point was very well illustrated by S.M. Low (1981) in her research on the meaning of the *nervios* category in Costa Rica, a category that takes on a specific meaning in this society but also in other Latin American cultures (Fainzang, 2000).

Research into the meaning of symptoms is also what has led some anthropologists to identify or define *culture-bound syndromes*, at the risk of producing or reinforcing stereotypes about ethnic specificities in this domain. Cathebras warns of this risk and pleads for the complex socio-medico-moral context in which a somatic complaint is expressed to be taken into account (see Cathebras, 2000). Analysis of the causal attributions and what they reveal about societies and cultures has also been carried out in the more general field of illness, where the study of symptoms is closely linked to that of the social etiology of illness (Fainzang, 1986; Jaffré, 1999), and where a certain number of nosological categories have been defined in relation to the symptoms associated with them.

Symptoms have also been studied from the point of view of their 'social function'. Honkasalo (1991) thus conceived of 'symptomisation' as a cultural coding of subjective sensations, serving to communicate a physical complaint, emotional problem or work conflict, and able to unify individuals in a social group and promote cohesion.

However, while the meaning of a symptom is socially acquired and culturally constructed, the act of bilaterally translating a symptom into a sign is not only the result of a collective construction. Onto this is superimposed an individual construction, nourished by the diverse influences exerted on the subjects and by their personal experience. A part of the symptom's meaning comes from this individual construction. This does not imply that this attribution of meaning is devoid of social underpinning and independent of a socio-cultural context, but rather that this construction differs depending on the individual, in relation to his/her personal history. Consequently, not only does this construction vary in accordance with the social and cultural context in which the subject lives (Kleinman, 1980; Alonzo, 1984; Sand Andersen, 2010), partly conditioning the meaning he/she attributes to a symptom – which is different from what a colleague, a neighbour or a cousin might attribute to an analogous symptom in his/her own body – but it is also susceptible to variation in the same subject at different periods of his/her life.

For their part, sociologists have examined the symptoms for which individuals consider it useful to take therapeutic action. The majority based their studies on symptoms as defined by biomedicine (Britten, 1994, 1996). In this they share a certain filiation with the works of Freidson (1984), who examined the variables that intervene in the process that leads laypeople to think they are ill and so decide to see a doctor. However we should note that Freidson did not dissociate the identification of a symptom with recourse to a doctor. For him it was case of identifying the criteria for which a bodily event represents a possible symptom of an illness and thus a reason for a consultation. Consequently he excluded cases where the sign is thought to be a symptom of an affliction that can be treated through self-medication. Or rather, when he mentioned self-medication, it was to refer to situations in which the person had an illness that was not recognised by the medical profession. He cited for example the *mal ojo* – the 'evil eye' for Latin Americans – for which individuals either treat themselves or go to see a traditional practitioner, since this is not a category recognised by biomedicine.

In the majority of these works, the perception of a symptom is conceived as the decisive element that leads to medical recourse, with particular attention paid to the type of recourse envisaged in accordance with the social environments. Barthe (1990) thus attempted to identify the differences between the 'upper' social groups and 'lower' social groups, and showed that, in line with Boltanski (1971), the perception of the seriousness of a symptom increases as one climbs the social hierarchy.

However, Aïach and Cèbe (1991) thought the opposite occurred: 'It is those who have a higher level' of knowledge about the body who are less inclined to pathologise their symptoms and 'hurry to the doctor's' (p. 73).

It is very clearly useful to reflect on the results of works examining the role of symptoms in therapeutic itineraries in the sense that these symptoms signal the point at which the subjects believe themselves to be ill. In this regard Barthe underlined the degree to which self-evaluation of a bodily event and its translation into pathological terms is a prerequisite for all decisions to seek care, whether self-administered or through medical consultation (Barthe, 1990). Nevertheless, because the appearance of a symptom does not necessarily lead to recourse to health professionals, we cannot deduce that the threshold for seeking care is identical when the subjects decide to manage the symptom by self-medication. The reasons and the conditions in which an individual considers a symptom to be pathological and in need of medical attention are not necessarily the same as the reasons and conditions in which he/she decides to manage a bodily sign through self-medication. The question of the link between the perception of a symptom and self-medication remains. Inversely however, some studies have concentrated more specifically on self-medication, independently from symptoms. This is the case for Raynaud (2008) who studied recourse to self-medication in relation to demographic, economic and social characteristics, and demonstrated their respective roles, as much in terms of the probability of resorting to self-medication as the modalities of the practice.

Yet, the operation in which the subjects decide to treat themselves partly relies on a process of decrypting a bodily sign which cannot be reduced to the same process that leads him/her to consult a doctor. The question is raised therefore as to the conditions in which the subjects decide to self-medicate when confronted with an ailment. At what point does a bodily sign become a symptom for him/her? And at what point does a symptom become a sign of the need to self-medicate rather than take recourse to a professional? The objective of this reflection is not so much to discover the symptoms that lead to self-medication, but the place the symptom occupies in the cognitive process leading to a decision to self-medicate. Here I will examine, based on material collected in the field,[1] the impact of bodily signs on the decision to treat oneself. I will show in this regard that the semiological controversy over the direction of the conversion between sign and symptom does not have much relevance in the context of self-medication, nor is the distinction between objective and subjective signs pertinent here. Examining the principal models on which the subject's choice to practice self-medication having identified a symptom are based will lead me instead to propose a distinction between absolute symptoms and relative symptoms.

Discussing 'construction' however does not entail considering that the symptom does not exist per se, that it is simply the result of a subjective perception, a fabrication by the subject, or even a product of his/her imagination. Equally, discussing identification does not involve denying the active dimension contained in the fact of turning a sign into a symptom, and consequently in the act of producing this symptom. It is therefore not a refusal of the concept of *construction* nor a belief that the symptom is necessarily an 'objective' phenomenon (as defined in medical semiology, in other words, as objectifiable by analysis, measures, markers, etc.), a phenomenon that the subjects would only be able to recognise or react to. The subjects can undertake the process of transforming a bodily sign into a symptom independently from whether the symptom is recognised as such by a health professional or not. From the moment they recognise or construct a bodily sign as a symptom it takes on an objective existence since it will then provoke a reaction, a response, and consequently a social practice – in this case self-medication. It is therefore more correct to discuss both the *construction* and the *identification* of symptoms. This would imply, anthropologically speaking, acknowledging the real existence of a symptom, independently of its medical reality (which is only another type of cultural construction). The construction and the identification should be considered as inextricable, since the symptom *exists* for the subjects at a given moment of their existence and it is this that induces them to choose to medicalise the sign they have perceived. Within the framework of self-medication, it is the subjects who produce an expertise, even if they are under multiple social and cultural influences; and it is the subjects who translate the bodily sign into a symptom. This operation cannot be reduced to simply interpreting the illness. It involves the subjects determining what the norm should apply to. It is the subjects' perception that makes the symptom exist, whether this corresponds or not with what a professional would first recognise as such, or with what the professional would consider as such if he/she was consulted.[2] The anthropological approach to our object only ascribes a reality to things that the subjects themselves do.

Between signs and symptoms

In medical semiology, the symptom is placed in opposition to the sign. The words 'symptom' and 'sign' are however used in diverse ways and are sometimes even interchangeable from one author to another. For some authors, a symptom is a particular species of sign. Peirce (1978) for example, sees the symptom as a 'subspecies' of the sign, in the sense that it is in a relationship vis-à-vis something else, to such an extent that it can be considered as if it is this other thing (cf. Sebeok, 1994). But a clinical sign cannot be identified as a symptom of an illness by only referring to the medical semiology code (Pouchain *et al.*, 1996; Ferreira, 2004). Consequently, a sign becomes a symptom through its clinical interpretation, whereas for other authors, it is the symptom that becomes a sign in the context of clinical discourse. For Shands (1970), tiredness is a symptom experienced by the patient, but the doctor notes it as a sign of impairment. Similarly, when Foucault (1963) wrote that the symptom 'is the form in which the disease presents itself' (p. 89), it is 'the intervention of a consciousness that transforms the symptom into a sign' (p. 92). Foucault noted that this operation, which gives the symptom the value of a signifying fact, is accomplished through comparison, recall and recording frequencies, simultaneities or successions: 'the symptom becomes […] a sign under a gaze receptive to the difference, the simultaneity or the succession, and to the frequency' (p. 93).

As we can see, the relationship between the terms 'sign' and 'symptom' varies, and it seems impossible to use these concepts in a consensual way when referring to the literature on the subject. In Barthes' (1985) proposition to bring together general and medical semiology, the concepts of symptoms and signs take on positions that are diametrically opposed to those given to them in Young's (1976) work. Barthes referred to Foucault to relate the symptom to the phenomenal and to conclude that it does not include a semiological dimension; for him it is 'a signifier not yet deciphered', while the sign is a symptom as it is placed in a description, and is the result of the doctor's organisational thinking. 'To go from a symptom to a sign is to go from the phenomenal to the semantic' (p. 274). However, for Young, signs are translated into symptoms in the sense that they are expressed and perceived in a socially acquired manner (Young 1976: 14–15).[3] This variation in usage appears even more pronounced when Sebeok (1994) considered 'subjective signs [to be] what the doctors wrongly label as signs' (p. 68).

However, whatever the direction in which these terms are linked in order to describe this process (from sign to symptom or from symptom to sign), it is striking to note that this transformation is only supposed to occur in the context of clinical discourse. Thus, Barthes (1972) believed that a symptom only becomes a sign when it enters into the context of clinical discourse, meaning when this transformation is performed by the doctor, and therefore through the mediation of language.

In truth, these various perspectives appear to be based on differing ways of comprehending the 'sign'. The sign is either perceived as a bodily sign, or as a clinical sign, so that, according to the authors, it either goes < sign → symptom > or < symptom → sign >. However, this transformation can also be performed by the subjects themselves;[4] and this is indeed what happens when they decide to take a given medicine from the medicine cabinet for a given symptom. Consequently, this transformation is realised through an intellectual operation that is also present in the process of self-medicating. For the subjects, these two schemes can coexist, and give rise to the following chain: < bodily sign → symptom → pathological sign >. Through a process of clinical self-examination and self-diagnosis, the sign (as a bodily sign) is converted into a symptom but the symptom in turn is converted into a sign of a pathological state and the need to medicalise it, an identification that is the result of a social process. Despite the usefulness of semiology in helping doctors convert signs and symptoms into diagnoses (Nessa, 1996), it is not certain in this regard whether these conceptual categories can genuinely contribute to our understanding of what leads a subject to medicalise a bodily event within the framework of self-medication. What is pertinent however from an anthropological point of view is that the relationship between sign and symptom depends on the level under examination, from the bodily level to the social one.

Moreover, the act of decoding a symptom (i.e. translating it into a sign) is not exclusively done by health professionals, even though it is generally assigned to medical expertise. The two registers (perceptive and cognitive) distinguished by Shands (1970) to account for the patient's activity *versus* the doctor's can be experimented with and drawn on by the same individual, and this is indeed what takes place in the context of self-medication. The symptoms can thus be of both a perceptive and a cognitive nature and constitute bodily events for the ill subject to understand, translate or interpret.

In these conditions, we cannot retain here the distinction between *subjective symptoms* – to refer to disorders perceived by the patient – and *objective symptoms* – to refer to disorders noted or measured by the doctor.[5] This distinction, collectively accepted by clinicians and developed within the framework of medical semiology, integrates another distinction also made by clinicians between *soft data* and *hard data*, to refer respectively to what the patients feel and what the doctors observe and measure (Sebeok, 1994). While these two categories of phenomena can clearly not be confused, this distinction is of little use in the context of self-medication. Indeed, individuals with autonomous subjectivity are not only, in Hunter's (2010) words, 'aware of and capable of acting on (their) choices for medical care', but their symptoms – which shape their actions and decisions – appear to them to be objective. The reality of the symptoms the subjects perceive renders, anthropologically speaking, the symptoms as objective as those considered as such by the doctors. From an anthropological point of view, the subjective signs are objective phenomena to the extent that they exist in the life and consciousness of the individuals and that they generate actions. Therefore, once it is constructed or identified as such, a symptom always has a reality that is *objective for the subject*. Such phrasing, which appears an oxymoron, is intended to affirm the objective reality of a subjective phenomenon from the moment that it induces a social practice, such as self-medication.

Symptoms and self-medication

The majority of the studies into the link between symptoms and self-medication agree that the most common symptom that individuals try to alleviate or cure is pain, that this is generally done by means of analgesics (Aïach and Cèbe, 1991; CSA/CECOP, 2007; Barthe, 1990; Buclin and Ammon, 2001; Burnier and Schneider, 2001; Burnier and Jeanneret, 2001; Queneau, 1999; Queneau et al., 2004; Molina, 1988; Steudler, 1999; Ferreira, 1994) and that analgesics are the family of medicines most frequently sold without a prescription.[6] However, knowing that pain is the main symptom for which subjects practice self-medication does not suffice in understanding the intellectual process that surrounds the identification of symptoms and dictates the response the subjects decide to make, from the discovery of a bodily sign up to self-medication via self-examination and self-diagnosis.

Clinical self-examination

Let us take the example of pain. The subjects undertake a clinical examination of themselves, by palpating their bodies, either seeking a reaction or a new pain in the area palpated or in order to uncover another symptom which is likely to then become additional proof of the existence of a pathology (Nylenna and Hjortdahl, 1987; Mol, 2003; Rice, 2008). In parallel with this sort of clinical self-examination, the subjects question themselves in the manner of a doctor: 'Have I eaten anything different from what I normally eat? Is there anything worrying me at the moment? Are there any particular reasons I might be "somatising?"'[7]

Here we can note the social dimension of the practice of self-examination. The very conditions in which it is practiced reveal something about the relationship the subjects have with those around them. The self-examination can be carried out in secret, either to avoid the reaction of a family member upon learning of the existence of the symptom which may lead him/her to urge the subject to see a doctor, or simply to avoid alarming him/her. The subjects thus explore their body and investigate the symptoms, away from prying eyes. But they may also want to keep quiet about the state of their body through embarrassment.[8] In this case, the self-examination can be carried out in bed, in the bathroom or in the toilets. The self-examination space is thus a private space, appropriate for an intimate clinical examination, when the subjects are not home alone.

Conversely, the self-examination can be carried out in front of everyone, in order to attract the attention or interest of family members. The subjects may add to this by complaining or verbalising the problem, leading the family to worry about their state of health. The aim is not necessarily to draw the secondary benefits of the 'sick role' (Mechanic, 1980) or what Brodwin (1994) calls the social performance of the pain or the symptoms in the context of chronic diseases, whether at home or in the workplace, in order to lighten one's workload. In fact, beyond the call for compassion, and aside from the fact that the dramatic nature of pain (in the Goffmanian sense of 'staging') can vary depending on the cultural tradition of the ill person,[9] the intention here is to solicit advice as to how to manage the symptom. The choice of the place in which to perform a clinical self-examination thus has social consequences since, in the first scenario, the subjects undertake the management of the problem alone and, in the second, they are no longer alone with the symptom and request the opinion of a third party, or even a collective decision.[10]

The self-examination can also bring to light what could be called 'symptoms of good health' that may counterbalance or negate the pathological character of a first symptom and prevent the subjects from medicalising it. When Richard (a 35-year-old computer specialist) had a stomach ache, he tried to identify it so as to treat it. He palpated his stomach in different places, worrying that he could have appendicitis. He was preparing to consult a doctor but when he pressed harder where the appendix is, he found no pain and he concluded that it could not be an appendicitis and that the pain was not serious, doubtless just the result of digestion problems. 'Feeling reassured', he 'did nothing'. In other words, he did not medicalise his pain.[11] Thus, during the clinical self-examination, symptoms also affect the cognitive work of the subjects by their absence, and can be conducive to modifying the original suppositions. While individuals tend to associate the absence of symptoms with the absence of illness (Errieau, 1987) in that the symptom is the ultimate element that objectifies the ailment in the subjects' eyes,[12] the presence or the absence of a second symptom however, discovered through a clinical self-examination, is likely to redirect the self-diagnosis.

From self-diagnosis to self-medication

When subjects feel pain or discover some other bodily sign, the meaning that they give it is likely to influence their practices of self-medication. Pain for example must first be interpreted before giving rise to the pharmaceutical response entailed in self-medication. The subjects try to interpret the pain by referring to events in their present life and to their past experience of perceiving such a symptom, and this guides how they choose to eliminate or contain it. In this way, not only does the translation of a bodily sign into a symptom depend on the context in which the patients find themselves and their history (what they are experiencing and have experienced before, the information they possess on the affliction, what they have previously identified as a symptom, their perception of the way health professionals have managed the problem in the past, etc.), but, in the context of self-medication, this translation mobilises a system of norms that may be specific to the subjects, leading them to choose to take a medicine after having analysed the context in which the symptom appears.

Mrs D for example interpreted a stomach ache as a pain linked to the imminence of her period because she was premenstrual, while Mr G interpreted this as an intestinal disorder because he had just come back from a trip abroad, whereas Miss F attributed it to a gastric pain following a copious meal in a restaurant. Or subjects may link the same symptom to a state of nerves, since they are at the point of accomplishing a social act that generates fear or emotion: a public presentation or performance, a medical examination, a romantic date, an exam, a competition, etc. Indeed, the same individual may attribute different meanings to the same pain, according to the point in time and the context in which it is experienced. Evidently such an attribution affects how subjects respond to the pain since, depending on the case, they may take an antispasmodic, an analgesic, an anti-inflammatory, an intestinal antiseptic or a tranquiliser. Then, beyond the specific sensory dimension of the symptom, when the medicine proves inefficacious for example, the subjects can be led to modify their interpretation of the pain if it persists when it should have stopped, or if it reappears later on. This may occur for example if a woman no longer has her period or if the social act involving strong emotions is over. For each interpretation the response will be specific and the pain management will be different.

The pain can be considered by the subjects either as a symptom of something else or as a problem to be treated in itself. Some try to treat it immediately by taking painkillers, while others resort to, as an alternative or a complement, other medicines they believe capable of treating the affliction for which the symptom is a sign, all the while observing the evolution of the symptom – or other symptoms that might provide information on the first one. Taking an anti-inflammatory to alleviate a pain previously diagnosed by a doctor (as for example a sign of arthritis) is not the same intellectual operation as taking an analgesic for an unknown pain while observing whether it diminishes or not, and whether other signs then accompany it, for example a new pain, in order to monitor its development and to confirm or deny the original diagnostic intuition. The appearance of a bodily event therefore presents a certain number of difficulties for the subjects who do not always know if they should consider it as a symptom of a pathology, as the pathology itself, or as one of its consequences. This goes for the stomach ache we used as an example above, which the subjects have some difficulty in interpreting straightaway in the semiological and diagnostic chain that they try to construct or reconstruct when faced with the affliction. The process of attributing a meaning to a bodily event is therefore not static. While individuals try to identify their symptom, they also observe its development, and in doing so extend the process of identification. After having put aside the hypothesis of appendicitis and since his stomach pains persisted, Richard decided to take an antispasmodic to alleviate them. But in addition to the pain, he experienced problems with his bowel functions for which he took a laxative. Since the pains persisted and the bowels problems returned after the treatment, this new occurrence of the affliction led him to a consultation, which resulted in a new diagnosis and a new treatment. This he then kept for a later date in order to self-medicate for the same symptom.

Indeed, it is the meaning assigned to a symptom that allows a prediction on its evolution, inciting a subject to self-medicate or not. Edith, a musician, who had been treated for breast cancer (and has since died from a brain tumour), lived in a village near to which ran a high-voltage power line. Since this worried her, she decided to become active in an ecological movement fearing she may develop another cancer. At the same time, the appearance of sleeping troubles and headaches, which she interpreted to be the result of the proximity of this power line,[13] led her to take tranquilizers and paracetamol, having little faith in the possibility of the symptoms disappearing on their own.

Individuals also carry out tests to which they assign a value of an experiment. For example, Denise, a 58-year-old speech therapist, had a sore throat following several past episodes of pharyngitis. 'I had repeated episodes of pharyngitis, with endless antibiotics prescribed by my GP; that weakened me, my intestines were weakened but it didn't sort out the problem.' During this new episode of the affliction, she went to the doctor again, but the doctor repeated the same antibiotic prescription which she refused to take. While her rejection of the antibiotic treatment was partly motivated by her conviction that it would not help since the pathology kept reappearing, it was also due to the new context in which this sore throat had appeared: an emotional break-up which 'shook' her and so she thought the symptom might be psychosomatic. On the advice of a friend, she decided to try a homeopathic treatment alongside throat lozenges but to no convincing effect. Since her sore throats continued, she discussed them with a colleague who explained that throat problems could be linked to sugar intolerance. So she decided to 'do an experiment'. She said: 'I bought a slab of chocolate to experiment with. I like chocolate a lot. So I ate all of it and my throat became very sore straight away.' She concluded that sugar was causing her recurrent sore throat. 'Sugar is one of life's sweetnesses,' she explained, 'it is difficult to accept having to go without, but I have got there now.' She linked her acceptance of going without the comfort of sugar to coming to terms with her sentimental disappointment and living without this 'sweetness'. From that point onwards, her choice of medicines taken by self-medication was carefully controlled in order to exclude any drug containing excess sugar.

Tijou Traoré's (2010) observation of diabetic patients revealed that they put medical information to the test by investigating the effects of consuming proscribed foods in order to test the relevance of the proscriptions concerning their daily habits. In contrast, Denise's experiment aimed to allow her to diagnose her pain in order to know how to manage the symptom. She assimilates this test with an experiment which, in this case, led to the demedicalisation of her symptom. Thus, unlike the act of choosing to take medicines out of habit because the subjects have these drugs at home or have been repeatedly prescribed them by their regular doctor, choosing or forsaking a medicine can thus result from a decision made after having conducted what is conceived as an experiment.

The construction/identification of a symptom raises the fundamental question of the distinction between the normal and the pathological. For Canguilhem (1966), the judgement regarding the pathological nature of a phenomenon is ultimately made by those who establish the norm. He wrote: 'in philosophy, we understand normative to be any judgement that assesses or qualifies a fact in relation to a norm, but this mode of judgement is fundamentally subordinated to the one who establishes the norm' (p. 77). But this locates the judgement in the register of expertise, or of medical authority. Yet, in the case of self-medication, it is the subjects who establish their own norm – be it superimposed or juxtaposed onto that established by medical discourse and/or onto that built by the pharmaceutical industry, or even onto that of those around them (family, social background, cultural environment, media), and consequently onto a norm in whose construction the social environment evidently plays a role. For example, Christiane experienced difficulty in getting to sleep after her husband left her. She discussed it with her mother who gave her a box of Stilnox[14] and suggested Christiane take one every evening as she herself did to manage her own insomnia. Based on her mother's advice, Christiane took this hypnotic, which she later replaced with Noctran[15] under the advice of a colleague, having decided that Stilnox did not have enough of an effect on her.

Evidently, the subjects also look for advice on the Internet, particularly when they are confronted with a symptom they do not recognise. For example, they seek advice on discussion forums to help them identify a symptom, discover its etiology and ascertain how serious it is (Akrich and Meadel, 2002). This was the case for Mrs F who one day experienced a very disagreeable strong bitter taste in her mouth and wanted to know whether this sensation was pathological and whether there was reason to be alarmed. We will return later to the information she obtained on the Internet on this subject (Chapter 4).

The operation undertaken is twofold since the person must first identify what he/she deems to be pathological, then ask him/herself whether this symptom is an indication that justifies self-medication. To examine the point at which a bodily sign becomes a symptom (or the point at which a symptom becomes a pathological sign) is, in the context of self-medication, to examine the criteria that transform a sign of a normal status into a sign of a pathological one, as well as the criteria that transform the status of the symptom from a sign needing treatment into a sign needing to be treated by *oneself*. Subsequently, it is not a case of simply referring to the medical norm to define what counts as pathological but of comparing this norm with what the subjects consider the norm in their own body. Thus, the subjects can recognise a bodily event as a phenomenon they have already seen or perceived (in their body or in someone else's) and whose occurrence can be followed or preceded by another symptom, in a sequence that takes a particular meaning. But they can also discover a sign for the first time and try to understand it. Germaine had a 'hazy voice'. She originally thought that it was a sign of aging and considered it normal. But she was troubled by her voice which she found rather disagreeable. She decided to suck sweets to soften it. But soon after, she found that people no longer recognised her on the telephone, which she thought odd, and the change in her voice then became pathological to her eyes. It is this designation that made her 'hazy voice' a symptom to be treated, in this case, a symptom of what she assumed to be pharyngitis.

Sometimes ailments are managed through self-medication because the doctor consulted does not agree with the subject in qualifying the bodily event as a symptom or in recognising the pathological nature of a symptom. This is the case for disorders that doctors qualify as 'functional', meaning symptoms not recognised as organic or physio-pathological (Cathebras, 2000), and for disorders sometimes referred to as 'medically unexplained symptoms' (Risor, 2010, 2011), a term that the patients often understand as a diplomatic way of telling them there is nothing wrong. But this is also the case when the subject develops a personal knowledge on the particular affliction experienced. Marie decided to treat her cephalgia herself because she thought she was not 'taken seriously' by her doctor. She had what she called '48-hour pain', a very severe headache which appeared several times a year and lasted 48 hours which she associated with 'stress at work'. Her doctor was sceptical and derisory when she told him about it; he retorted in a mocking tone that it did not exist and that the problem was 'in her head'. She considered her headache to be an authentic pathological entity, with the same manifestation, intensity and duration every time. Thus, she decided to treat it on her own from then on: 'I know what it is. In my case, this headache means I am too stressed at work. I know myself. I know what I need,' she said. When the pain comes, she takes high doses of anti-inflammatories for 48 hours.

For similar reasons Edith, mentioned above, self-medicated to treat her insomnia and cephalgia. Doubting the reassuring information provided by the public authorities and the assessment they support that high-voltage power lines are not harmful, Edith, who nurtured a fear of developing cancer because of her exposure to electromagnetic fields, spoke to her doctor about her sleeping troubles and her headaches. Having been told that it was just her anxiety causing the problem, she decided, alone, to take tranquilisers to combat her insomnia. Sometimes, subjects are led to decide to take a medicine after recognising a symptom they think they have had when reading the pharmaceutical leaflet, without necessarily looking at that point in time for a medicine to manage the ailment. Françoise regularly tidies her domestic pharmacy in order to discard drugs that are past their sell-by date. Not remembering the indications of one of the medicines she found (a medicine prescribed some time before for her husband), she opened the box and read the pharmaceutical leaflet to see if it could ever be useful and check if it was worth keeping. She then recognised a symptom she occasionally experienced (nausea) and said: 'But yes, that is something I get! I will take that the next time I get my "sea sickness"' (a term she uses to refer metaphorically to the sensation these nauseas give her). This process is thus the opposite of that which consists of looking for a remedy to a symptom, since here, finding the medicine precedes the search for an appropriate medicine for an identified symptom.

We can see the extent to which the symptom is a structuring element of the practice of self-medication. The denomination itself of the ailment is often based on the symptom or on one of its characteristics. The subjects engage in a sort of self-nosography, a denomination constructed in reference to the bodily sign itself (for example the 'hazy voice'), or to a characteristic of the symptom such as its duration (the '48-hour pain'), or even to what it evokes metaphorically (the 'sea-sickness'). In opposition to the descriptive or metaphorical denomination ('my 48-hour pain') is the causal or etiological denomination (such as 'my intolerance to sugar'), which serve as categories allowing future reference to the ailment.

If, in the context of a medical consultation, the medicine confirms the illness in the eyes of the patient in that the prescription attests its necessity (Dagognet, 1996; Whyte *et al.* 2002), it also confirms the illness by its effects (Nichter and Vuckovic, 1994). This is what takes place not only when the subjects use a medicine for *therapeutic* ends, a use which allows them to verify de facto the efficacy of a medicine, but also when they use a medicine for *diagnostic* ends. Thus, Hubert took an intestinal antiseptic to see if his 'upset' was caused by a 'stomach bug'. It is not only the identification of a symptom that leads to a choice of medicine, but the taking of a medicine itself can be intended to allow an identification of the ailment. Thus, Monique, when faced with a cough she could not explain since it was not associated with a sore throat, which would have made her consider pharyngitis, took antihistamines to see if her cough would go away. For her it was not simply a case of alleviating or eradicating the cough but of identifying it and making a diagnosis. If the drug had worked, she would have concluded that it was an allergic cough. Here, the medicine is used as a diagnostic tool as well as an attempt to cure the affliction. Since the antihistamines had no effect, she then considered whether it would be appropriate to take an antibiotic treatment to see if it was an infection. The use of antibiotics here did not follow a diagnosis; rather, it preceded it. Unlike the mechanism underpinning what Lakoff (2006) called 'pharmaceutical reason' where, in contemporary biomedical psychiatry, it is in relation to the treatment to which it responds that illness is *defined*, here, it is as a result of the medicine to which the symptom responds that the illness is *diagnosed*. Nichter and Vuckovic (1994) described this diagnostic technique, highlighting the fact that: 'Medications play a direct role in the process of diagnosis when practitioners identify an illness on the basis of treatment response.' In this case however, the identification is not done by health professionals, but by the subjects themselves.

Absolute symptoms and relative symptoms

If we believe Sebeok (1994), the relationship between sign and symptom is obvious to the doctor, and a given symptom corresponds necessarily and consequently to a specific illness. He wrote on this subject: 'a symptom is a compulsive, automatic, non-arbitrary sign, such that the signifier is coupled with the signified in the manner of a natural link' (p. 46). In fact, this can also occur in the context of self-medication. Even though the same symptom can signify diverse illnesses and even though the same illness can present different symptoms, the subjects can sometimes establish a one-to-one relationship between the two for their own case, modelled on medical semiology. They can link a symptom to an illness and thus infer a diagnosis, or a provisional one at least, in conformity with Sebeok's description of medical semiological activity, or with what Jaffré (1999) qualified as symptoms of monosemic interpretation. However, as Umberto Eco (1992) highlighted, the meaning of a sign is not invariably unequivocal. A symptom is always identified in relation to a precise context.

Yet, not only is the translation of a bodily sign into a symptom not identical from one person to another (on the model of 'in my case, it means that'), but it is not necessarily identical for the same person from one point in his/her life to another, as we saw with Denise, who modified both the interpretation and the management of her sore throat when a change happened in her life, in this case a break-up. Consequently, while there can be an automatic relationship between sign and symptom, a symptom can also take a specific meaning which is only valid for a given individual in a sort of idiosyncratic nosography. Therefore, in contrast to the usual approach of anthropologists to therapeutic strategies in a given cultural environment, which is generally in reference to a collective norm (expressing that of the dominant system of thought), here we have a recourse to medicines that is based on a norm nourished by both a collective norm and an individual one, created from the subjects' experience and the different influences that are exerted on them, and resulting in the attribution of variable values to the same symptom.

Consequently, the process of decoding a symptom lies at the intersection of the individual and the collective. The interpretation of a symptom is simultaneously individual and collective to the extent that it is both *typical* of a society,[16] a cultural group or a social environment, and *specific* to a subject. To say it is 'individual' does not mean that this attribution of meaning can be defined as psychological. As individual as it may be in that it is anchored in a personal history, this construction rests on the cultural representations and logics it is founded on. Discussing individual construction emphasises the subjects' personal experience, which, though inseparable from the social context in which they live, should be envisaged in its singularity. Thus the meaning the subject assigns to a symptom will be different from that which another subject would assign to a similar symptom in his/ her own body. Indeed, although the appearance of a symptom can be differently perceived depending on the social context in which it appears and depending on the social background of the subject (Barthe, 1990), assimilating a subject simply into his/her social environment would be reductive, even when the other sociodemographic variables such as age and gender are taken into account. This would not only amount to neglecting the personal history of the subject but also to unifying his/her history as if it is invariable. Subjects react differently to a symptom depending on whether they have already experienced it, whether they have obtained supplementary information on it or not, whether they know someone who has already experienced it or not, whether they have consulted the Internet on this subject or not, whether they have consulted a doctor for an analogous symptom in the past or not, whether this symptom was cured, alleviated or followed by other symptoms, etc. In a sense, at every moment of the subject's life, the context in which the symptom appears is different. Consequently, while we can accept Sebeok's (1994) view that symptoms are not arbitrary signs, their meaning is not for all that automatic. They take on a relative value because of the fact that they can take on a given value for a given individual, not only distinct from that of another person, but also distinct from the value they could take at another moment in the history of this individual. There is thus a tension in the symptom's interpretation between the new conditions of its appearance and the idiosyncratic doctrines forged by the subjects regarding it.

While, as we have seen, opposing subjective signs and objective signs makes no sense for the subject practising self-medication, in contrast, a pertinent distinction is noticeable between symptoms with an absolute value and symptoms with relative value. By virtue of this, we should distinguish between the value that people attribute to a symptom as a result of their medical knowledge, their socialisation, their culture (Kleinman, 1980; Kirmayer, Young and Robbins, 1994; Hagberg, 1995) public health messages, explanations received from doctors or pharmaceutical leaflets,[17] etc., and the value they attribute to a symptom in reference to themselves, their own bodies and their own histories.

Indeed, there are symptoms of 'absolute value' when a given sign necessarily takes a given value or meaning that is valid for all, but there are also symptoms of 'relative value' when a sign takes a specific value that is only valid for the subject. The coexistence of symptoms with absolute value and those with relative value results from the tension between the collective and individual dimensions of the task of decoding symptoms that is carried out in the context of self-medication. This coexistence is what makes that process of constructing and/or identifying symptoms, undertaken by the subjects, an authentic semiological process.

Notes

1 Although web users comprehensively describe their symptoms and their therapeutic decisions on the various discussion forums available on the web, where social scientists today concentrate much of their investigations (Akrich and Méadel, 2004; Hardey, 2004), there are only a very few observations of the concrete practices in this area available.
2 If the subject has a fever but does not notice it or pays little attention to it and so takes no action (notably medicinal) against it, this circumstance will not be retained within the framework of this study in that the subject must develop a discourse or a practice concerning a bodily event for the fact to become pertinent.
3 My use of the term symptom is closer to Young's, to the extent that the sign, the thing that is perceived, acquires here the status of a symptom once it is considered to be pathological.
4 As Massé (1999b) underlined in his 'semiotic study of psychological distress', the symptom, before becoming a clinical sign, is a sign for the ill person and his/her family.
5 And consequently take the value of a 'sign', at least in the terminology of authors such as Foucault (1963) or Shands (1970).
6 This has recently been confirmed by a research project, carried out on 8,000 people by questionnaire over the telephone. It showed that the main symptoms for which people take recourse to self-medication are headaches, migraines, lumbago, influenza, colds, period pains and dental pain (SFETD seminar entitled 'Douleur et automédication', 6 October 2009, Paris).
7 A common way in French of saying the trouble may be psychosomatic.
8 This embarrassment can also indeed prevent the subject from consulting a doctor for the symptom.
9 On the cultural dimension of the expression of symptoms and complaints, see Zborowski (1952) who demonstrated the cultural components of reactions to pain, and Zola (1966) who highlighted the way in which different 'ethnocultural' groups, notably Americans of Italian or Irish origin, express their complaints.
10 It should be noted that the tendency to manage an affliction in an individual or collective way is also linked to other mechanisms, and in this case cultural habits (cf. Fainzang, 2001b).
11 We will return to his case and its progression later.
12 Even though the equivalence between symptom and illness can be the object of divergent assessments, as in the case of allergy (cf. Raffaetà, 2011; Champaloux, 2006).
13 An interpretation that is in fact backed up by the conclusions of some studies: 'People living near high-voltage or very high-voltage power lines have more health problems such as sleeping disorders, memory and hearing loss, as well as headaches, irritability and depressive states. These symptoms diminish significantly when they leave the area affected by the high-voltage line.' (www.psychomedia.qc.ca/sante/2008-03-22/lignes-a-haute-tension-cancers-maux-de-tete-depression).
14 A hypnotic containing Zolpidem.
15 A drug that combines several active ingredients.
16 Such as the 'crise de foie' syndrome for example (Pouchelle, 2007).
17 We will further examine the different sources of knowledge in chapter 4.

References

Aïach P. and Cèbe D., 1991, *Expression des symptômes et conduites de maladie*, Paris: Editions de l'Inserm/Doin.
Akrich M. and Méadel C., 2002, 'Prendre ses médicaments / prendre la parole: les usages des médicaments par les patients dans les listes de discussion électroniques', *Sciences Sociales et Santé*, 20, 1 (special issue: 'Les médicaments : des prescriptions aux usages'): 89–116.

Akrich M.,and Méadel C., 2004, 'Problématiser la question des usages', *Sciences Sociales et Santé* 22, 1 (special issue: 'Les technologies de l'information à l'épreuve des pratiques'): 5–20.

Alonzo A.A., 1984, 'An illness behaviour paradigm: a conceptual exploration of a situational-adaptation perspective', *Social Science and Medicine*, 19, 5: 499–510.

Barthe J.F., 1990, 'Connaissance profane des symptômes et recours thérapeutiques', *Revue française de sociologie*, XXXI, 2 : 283–296.

Barthes R., 1972, 'Sémiologie et médecine', in: R. Bastide (ed.), *Les sciences de la folie*, Paris: Mouton : 37–46.

Barthes R., 1985, *L'aventure sémiologique*, Paris: Le Seuil.

Boltanski L., 1971, 'Les usages sociaux du corps', *Annales*, 1: 205–231.

Britten N., 1994, 'Patients' ideas about medicines. A qualitative study in a general practice population', *British Journal of General Practice*, 44: 465–468.

Britten N., 1996, 'Lay views of drugs and medicines: orthodox and unorthodox accounts', in: S.J. Williams, and M. Calnan (eds), *Modern medicine. Lay perspectives and experiences*, London: UCL Press.

Brodwin P.E., 1994, 'Symptoms and Social Performances: the case of Diane Reden', in: M.-J. DelVecchio Good, P.E. Brodwin, B.J. Good and A. Kleinman (eds) *Pain as human experience. An anthropological perspective.*, Berkeley: University of California Press, 77–99.

Buclin T. and Ammon C. (eds), 2001, *L'automédication: pratique banale, motifs complexes*, Genève: Médecine et Hygiène, Cahiers Médico-Sociaux, 11–29.

Burnier M. and Schneider M.P., 2001, 'De l'automédication à la non-observance thérapeutique', in: T. Buclin and C. Ammon (eds), *L'automédication: pratique banale, motifs complexes*, Genève: Médecine et Hygiène, Cahiers Médico-Sociaux, 89–97.

Burnier M.J. and Jeanneret O., 2001, 'L'automédication, une pratique en quête de sens: sa place dans le self care et la promotion de la santé', in: T. Buclin and C. Ammon (eds), *L'automédication: pratique banale, motifs complexes*, Genève: Médecine et Hygiène, Cahiers Médico-Sociaux, 11–29.

Canguilhem G., 1966, *Le normal et le pathologique*, Paris: PUF.

Cathebras P., 2000, 'Douleur, somatisation et culture: peut-on aller au-delà des stéréotypes?', *Douleur et analgésie*, 13, 3: 159–162.

Champaloux B., 2006, *Une approche anthropologique des maladies allergiques des enfants*, ATC Environnement–santé, Inserm/Ministère de la recherche, October 2006.

CSA/CECOP, 2007, 'Les Français et l'automédication', enquête exclusive réalisée pour la Mutualité Française.

Dagognet F., 1996, *Pour une philosophie de la maladie*, Paris: Ed. Textuel.

DelVecchio Good M.J., Brodwin P.E., Good B.J., Kleinman A., (eds), 1994, *Pain as human experience. An anthropological perspective*, Berkeley: University of California Press.

Eco U., 1992, *La production des signes*. Paris: Le livre de Poche.

Errieau G., 1987, 'La prescription au quotidien', *Prospective et santé*, 43: 63–66.

Fainzang S., 1986, *'L'intérieur des choses'. Maladie, divination et reproduction sociale chez les Bisa du Burkina*. Paris: L'Harmattan.

Fainzang S., 2000, *Of malady and misery. An Africanist perspective of illness in Europe*, Amsterdam: Het Spinhuis Publishers (Coll. Health, Culture and Society).

Fainzang S., 2001b, *Médicaments et société. Le patient, le médecin et l'ordonnance*, Paris: Presses Universitaires de France.

Ferreira J., 1994, 'O Corpo Sígnico: uma perspectiva antropológica', in: P.C. Alves and C.S. Minayo (eds), *Saúde e Doença: um olhar antropológico*, Rio de Janeiro: Fiocruz.

Ferreira J., 2004, *Soigner les mal-soignés. Ethnologie d'un centre de soins gratuits*, Paris: L'Harmattan, Coll. Logiques sociales.

Foucault J-P., 1963, *Naissance de la Clinique. Une archéologie du regard médical*, Paris: Presses Universitaires de France.

Friedson E., 1984, *La profession médicale*. Paris: Payot ('Médecine et sociétés').

Good B.J. and M.-J. Delvecchio-Good, 1981, 'The meaning of symptoms: a cultural hermeneutic model for clinical practice', in: L. Eisenberg and A. Kleinman (eds), *The relevance of social science for medicine*, Dordrecht/Boston/Lancaster: D. Reidel Publishing Company, 165–196.

Hagberg S., 1995, 'Cultural variations in symptom attribution', *Canadian Journal of Psychiatry*, 40, 5: 275–6.

Hardey M., 2004, 'Internet et société: reconfigurations du patient et de la médecine?', *Sciences sociales et santé*, 22, 1: 5–20.

Hay M.C., 2008, 'Reading sensations: understanding the process of distinguishing `fine' from 'sick'', *Transcultural Psychiatry*, 45, 2: 198–229.

Honkasalo M.-L., 1991, 'Medical symptoms: a challenge for semiotic research', *Semiotica*, 87, ¾: 251–268.

Hunter, N.D., 2010, 'Rights talk and patient subjectivity: the role of autonomy, equality and participation norms'. *Georgetown Law Faculty Publications and Other Works*. Paper 473. [http://scholarship.law.georgetown.edu/facpub/473].

Jaffré Y., 1999 : 'La maladie et ses dispositifs', in: Y. Jaffré and J.P. Olivier de Sardan (eds), *La construction sociale des maladies*, Paris: Les Presses universitaires de France (Collection : Les champs de la santé), 41–68.

Kirmayer L.J., Young A. and Robbins J.M., 1994, 'Symptom attribution in cultural perspective', *Canadian Journal of Psychiatry*, 39, 10: 584–95.

Kleinman A., 1980, *Patients and healers in the context of culture*, Berkeley: University of California Press.

Kleinman A., 2002, 'Santé et stigmate", *Actes de la recherche en sciences sociales*, 3, 143: 97–99.

Lakoff A., 2006, *Pharmaceutical reason. Knowledge and value in global psychiatry*, Cambridge: Cambridge University Press (Series: Cambridge Studies in Society and the Life Sciences).

Low S.M., 1981, 'The meaning of nervios: a sociocultural analysis of symptom presentation in San Jose, Costa Rica', *Culture, Medicine and Psychiatry*, 5, 1: 25–47.

Martinez-Hernáez, A., 2000, *What's behind the symptom? On psychiatric observation and anthropological understanding*. Amsterdam: Harwood Academic Publishers.

Massé R., 1999b, 'Les conditions d'une anthropologie sémiotique de la détresse psychologique', *Recherche sémiotique/Semiotic Inquiry*, 19, 1: 39–62.

Mechanic D., 1980, 'The experience and reporting of common physical complaints', *Journal of Health and Social Behavior*, 21: 146–155.

Mol A.-M., 2003, *The body multiple: Ontology in medical practice*, Durham: Duke University Press.

Molina N., 1988, *L'automédication*, Paris: PUF (Coll: Les champs de la santé).

Nessa J., 1996, 'About signs and symptoms: Can semiotics expand the view of clinical medicine?' *Theoretical Medicine and Bioethics*, 17, 4: 363–377.

Nichter M. and Vuckovic N., 1994, 'Agenda for an anthropology of pharmaceutical practice', *Social Science and Medicine*, 39, 11: 1509–1525.

Nylenna M. and Hjortdahl P., 1987, 'How do patients evaluate cancer related symptoms and signs? A study from general practice', *Scand J Prim Health Care*, 5: 117–122.

Peirce C.S., 1978, *Écrits sur le signe*, Paris: Seuil.

Pouchain D., Attali C., de Butler J., Clément G., Gay B., Molina J., Olombel P. and Rouy J.-L., 1996, *Médecine générale. Concepts et pratique*, Paris: Masson.

Pouchelle M.-C., 2007, 'La crise de foie : une affection française ?', *Terrain*, 48: 149–164.

Queneau P., 1999, 'Automédication en antalgiques', in: P. Queneau (ed.), *Automédication, autoprescription, autoconsommation*, Paris: John Libbey, 84–95.

Queneau P., Froudarakis M., Salvador M, Villani P. and Vital-Durand D., 2004, 'Automédication concernant les antalgiques", in: P. Queneau and G. Ostermann (eds), *Le médecin, le malade et la douleur*. Paris: Masson, 389–398.

Raffaetà R. 2011, 'The allergy epidemic, or when medicalisation is bottom-up', in: S. Fainzang and C. Haxaire (eds), *Of bodies and symptoms. Anthropological perspectives on their social and medical treatment*, Tarragona: URV Publicacions, 59–77.

Raynaud D., 2008, 'Les déterminants du recours à l'automédication', *Revue Française des Affaires sociales*, 1: 81–94.

Rice T., 2008, 'Noisy hearts: auto-auscultation and sound in illness experience', Biennial EASA Conference: 'Experiencing diversity and mutuality', Ljubljana.

Risor M.B., 2010, 'Healing and recovery as a social process among patients with medically unexplained symptoms (MUS)', in: S. Fainzang, H.E. Hem and M.B. Risor (eds), *The Taste for Knowledge: medical anthropology facing medical realities,* Copenhagen: Aarhus University Press, 133–149.

Risor M.B., 2011, 'The process of symptomization. Clinical encounters with functional disorders', In: S. Fainzang and C. Haxaire (eds), *Of bodies and symptoms. Anthropological perspectives on their social and medical treatment*, Tarragona: URV Publicacions, 21–37.

Sand Andersen R., 2010, 'Anthropological perspectives on the biomedically defined problem of "patient delay"', in: S. Fainzang, H.E. Hem and M.B. Risor (eds), *The taste for knowledge: medical anthropology facing medical realities*, Copenhagen: Aarhus University Press, 57–68.

Sebeok T.A., 1994 (1921), *Signs. An introduction to semiotics*. Toronto/Buffalo/London: University of Toronto Press.

Shands H.C., 1970, *Semiotic approaches to psychiatry*, The Hague: Mouton.

Steudler F., 1999, 'Aspects sociologiques de l'automédication', in: P. Queneau (ed), *Automédication, autoprescription, autoconsommation*. Paris, John Libbey, 23–32.

Tijou Traoré A., 2010, 'L'expérience dans la production de savoirs profanes sur le diabète chez les patients diabétiques à Bamako (Mali)', *Sciences Sociales et Santé*, 28, 4: 41–76.

Whyte S.R., Van der Geest S. and Hardon H., 2002, *Social lives of medicines*, Cambridge, Cambridge University Press (coll. studies in medical anthropology).

Young A., 1976, 'Some implications of medical beliefs and practices for social anthropology', *American Anthropologist*, 78: 5–24.

Zborowski M., 1952, 'Cultural components in response to pain', *J Soc Issues* 8: 16–30.

Zola I.K., 1966, 'Culture and symptoms. An analysis of patients' presenting complaints', *Amer. Sociol. Rev.* 31: 615–30.

3 Cultural and practical reasons[1]

Despite the fact that pharmacy sales figures in France show a lower use of self-medication compared to other European countries (Lecomte, 1994; Karsenty, 1994; Blenkisopp and Bradley, 1996; Burnier and Schneider, 2001; Burnier and Jeanneret, 2001; Coulomb and Baumelou, 2007), the practice of self-medication is not new.[2] Numerous works in fact have already taken an interest in the practice and endeavoured to define its factors in accordance with the socioeconomic or socioprofessional characteristics of the users and depending on the pathologies concerned (Molina, 1988; Barthe, 1990; Aïach and Cèbe, 1991; Buclin and Ammon, 2001; Raynaud, 2008).[3] The effect of social background on recourse to self-medication is in truth a rather controversial aspect in these works, as noted in my discussion of the influence of this factor on the perception of symptoms. Thus, McKinlay (1975) observed a greater tendency to self-medicate amongst poor people and those belonging to the lower social classes; whereas Raynaud (2008) showed that it was more common for people of working age, in good health and from more privileged social and cultural backgrounds to treat themselves without any prior advice or by following pharmacists' recommendations, while people from more modest backgrounds took less recourse to self-medication and more often followed the advice of a doctor when they did so.

The literature, both medical and sociological, has shown the practical and economic dimensions of motivations for self-medication (Molina, 1988; Thoër *et al.,* 1988; Lecomte, 1988; Laure, 1998; Karsenty, 2009). These studies emphasise the point that the decision to self-medicate is often made in order to save time and money. Thoër *et al.* (1988) thus noted that self-medication is frequently used to treat health problems the patients consider to be benign, for which they think it unnecessary to consult a doctor, and for chronic problems that the individuals have learnt to manage autonomously, and that as such self-medication is considered as a means of gaining time and money. It is a case of eliminating the waiting period that would be required to get an appointment or in the waiting room on the day, or even to avoid the costs involved in a consultation that could result in being prescribed medicines that are not for a large part eligible for reimbursement, or caused by what Raynaud (2008) refers to as the 'opportunity cost' of the consultation. The term 'impatient patient' is sometimes used to account for this aspect of self-medication.[4] The desire to treat oneself more quickly is indeed reinforced by the significant waiting times in contemporary France linked to problems with the medical demographic – difficulties that are likely to be exacerbated in the near future. The development of self-medication is also the result of public policies and professional practices, such as, for example, the removal of eligibility for reimbursement from a growing number of medicines and the fact that many doctors charge over the standard fees.[5]

In truth it is difficult to determine the economic advantages and disadvantages this practice represents for the consumer and, in any case, the users themselves have trouble answering this question. Indeed, for some patients, the removal of eligibility for reimbursement from numerous medicines is an advantage in that it renders their prescription unnecessary and in consequence the medical consultation also becomes unnecessary. However, on the other hand, some users see it as a financial obstacle to self-medication and say they do not understand the economic logic of the drug policy. Emile thus noticed that a tube of antifungal ointment that costs 5.20€ when prescribed by a doctor was sold to him for 9.50€ when he wanted to buy it without a prescription even though the two tubes contain the same molecule (terbafine hydrochloride) in the same proportions. Consequently, he remains doubtful of the savings that self-medication is supposed to allow him to make. For his part, Lionel (a 55-year-old printer) refuses to self-medicate when it means he has to pay more for a medicine. He does not understand why he should pay for something he believes he is being unfairly charged for, since this purchase in self-medication means the public health insurance fund saves on the fee of the consultation avoided.

However, saving time or money is not the only factor in the subject's decision as to whether to practice self-medication. Beyond the economic aspects, self-medication involves a certain relationship with the body and with medicines but also with medical authority. This relationship is based both on the personal experience of the ill subject and on the image he/she has built of the practice, which itself is linked to its image in the social space, since as we have seen, the fact that the public authorities encourage self-medication today means that it is now losing its deviant character.[6] The subjects now know that their 'capacity' to treat themselves has been recognised in some circumstances, i.e. 'in benign situations' or 'for benign pathologies', as the official documents on the subject make clear. It is in fact under such conditions that, in questionnaire-based studies on the subject, the respondents claimed to only practice self-medication (DGS/CSA-TMO, 2002), leading the majority of authors to conclude that the practice mainly concerns the 'minor ailments of daily life' (Laure, 1998; Raynaud, 2008). The most common reasons mentioned by these works are problems that are not serious enough to trouble a doctor with, or ones that only need the advice of a pharmacist, or again ailments the subjects already know well enough to treat themselves (Saubadu, 1988). The Afipa-Sofres inquiry in 2001 (DGS/CSA-TMO, 2002) revealed that the biggest reason for self-medication is the need for fast relief; following this is the fact that the problem is considered as benign or that it is a familiar problem for which the medicine is already known.

Reasons and reasoning

My preliminary investigations partly corroborated the results of these works: not surprisingly people reported, at least at the start of the interviews, their decisions to *take recourse to* self-medication in cases of minor benign ailments, and often claimed to *limit this recourse* to benign situations only.[7] Self-medication is often practiced as a repetition of a previous prescription – the subjects base their actions on the competence of a professional and reproduce the diagnosis and treatment proposed, thinking there is no need to consult a second time for a symptom believed to be similar and to which they attribute an identical etiology to that of the doctor consulted in the past. Let us recall Richard's case, whose stomach pains, which he originally judged to be of no importance and did not medicalise, he subsequently treated with an antispasmodic; then, when he also experienced transit disorder, he took a laxative. But since the pains did not go away and the constipation and bloating continued after the treatment was over, he resolved to consult a doctor fearing an intestinal occlusion. The doctor declared that his colic was caused by stress and prescribed tranquilisers. As this new episode resulted in a new diagnosis and a new treatment, this is what he will select to self-medicate when faced with the same symptom in the future. Now, when he has stomach pains, he no longer consults a doctor ('Now, I know there's no point in going to the doctor's when I get that,' he explained), because he thinks he is capable of managing his pains, to which he attributes the same etiology and the same therapy from then on, by taking tranquilisers. We will see in this regard that the subjects extend the concept of 'benign' and that, along with how they construct their knowledge on medicines, this leads them to self-medicate in situations where the benignity is clearly debatable.

Self-medication can also be linked to a form of modesty or embarrassment which, we have seen, can organise the modalities of clinical self-examination, away from prying eyes of the family, reluctant to any performance of the symptoms (Brodwin, 1994; Delecchio-Good et al., 1994; Nichter and Vuckovic, 1994). But this also sometimes underpins the reluctance to consult a doctor. This is the case for Mrs V who suffers from recurring haemorrhoids but said she is very uncomfortable discussing this affliction with a doctor, fearing he/she may want to examine her (she talked about this as 'shame'): 'For things like haemorrhoids I go to the pharmacy to buy what I need; this type of examination by a doctor bothers me, I am a bit ashamed.' This is also the case for Hervé, a 50-year-old business manager, who suffers from recurring genital herpes but does not want to consult a doctor about it. He explained that he 'didn't want to let them fiddle with his pecker for that', and even bought acyclovir online to avoid going to the pharmacy and having to mention the problem in front of everyone, or let people to guess what it is. This self-medication is thus a secret, intimate practice. Self-medication also provides a means to avoid worrying a family member, as we saw for clinical self-examination, even when the illness in question does not require any sort of bodily examination. The desire to hide this recourse influences the practical modalities of self-medication. For example, Evelyne takes tranquilisers in secret (by way of a hypnotic) so as not to worry her mother who would be alarmed if she found out that her daughter has trouble sleeping. Hidden self-medication aims to avert the reaction of a family member who may get upset or urge the subject to consult a doctor on discovering the existence of the problem. Likewise, Mr D, who at times suffers from anxiety linked to his marital relations, does not want to consult a doctor on the subject for fear of getting caught in a cycle of medical care and a regular and onerous prescription of psychoactive drugs. He discovered the presence of tranquilisers at his father's house and started to steal a few Temesta pills from time to time during his visits from his father's domestic pharmacy, which he occasionally self-administered to relieve his anxiety.

Nevertheless, the reasons for which subjects practice self-medication, such as familiarity with the medicine or the benign nature of the affliction, coexist with other motives (Good and Delvecchio-Good, 1981; Lemoigne, 1999; Steudler, 1999; Ostermann, 1999; Queneau, 1999; Queneau et al., 2004; Collin, Ottero and Monnais, 2006; Nouguez, 2007; Sarradon-Eck et al., 2007). By resituating accounts of self-medication in their specific contexts (taking into account the previous episodes of occurrence of the affliction in question, the recourse this gave rise to, the resulting events, etc.), it becomes clear that other rationalities are also at work. Here in fact, my research highlights other aspects of this recourse that relate to the judgement and critical assessment of medical work.

Indeed, it is sometimes, inversely, a conviction that the GP would not be able to manage the affliction that discourages some people from seeking a consultation – a conviction rooted in past experience. The decision to self-medicate is therefore defensive, brought about by previously experienced misfortune following recourse to a doctor.

A disappointing experience

To illustrate this point, I will return to the case of Germaine and her 'hazy voice', which she considered to be pathological from the point when people no longer recognised her on the telephone. Thinking she had pharyngitis, she then tried to stem the problem with 'throat syrups' but to no effect. Soon after, she had a fever and so she decided to consult her GP. After examining her throat, the doctor declared that there was nothing there, but since she had a fever she probably had sinusitis causing an irritation and he prescribed her antibiotics, which she took scrupulously. When the treatment was over, her voice was identical to before and she still had a fever. So she consulted a different doctor who referred her for a blood test. On reading her results, he noted a fall in her immunity and concluded her problem was 'viral' and that the only option was to 'wait for it to pass'. She finally decided to consult an otorhinolaryngologist on her own initiative who detected an oedema linked to oesophageal refluxes. The failure of her previous consultations had convinced her to treat herself thereafter, or otherwise to consult a specialist directly.

Similarly, Denise chooses to self-medicate when she has a sore throat. Her reluctance to consult a doctor originated in the fact that her doctor had prescribed her 'endless antibiotics' which 'weakened' her and made her intestines more 'fragile', without however 'solving the problem'. 'So now I try to treat myself alone. A friend advised me to use gentler methods, and little by little I have got there.' Now, she only consults her doctor on rare occasions, even though she is not systematically hostile to allopathy.[8] She only consults for afflictions she is not able to understand and control or which worry her particularly, such as when she felt 'shooting pains in her eyes' which worried her: 'Then, I didn't try to treat myself with eyewash or something like that. I went to a doctor immediately because I had a grandmother who was almost blind, and my father had glaucoma, so I am careful!' An individual's decision to consult a doctor or not is largely dependent on his/her personal and family history. But recourse to self-medication is for Denise the result of unsuccessful consultations.

For her part, Chantal, a 68-year-old retired teacher, recounted:

> One day, I had very severe stomach pain. I called a doctor who put ice on my stomach. But the pain didn't go away. So I decided to go to the hospital, to the gastroenterology department. There, they did some examinations and they discovered a tumour as big as a grapefruit which had burst. They operated on me and discovered a load of cysts on my ovaries!

Since then, Chantal avoids consulting a GP and looks for other solutions: 'So I'd rather go directly to the hospital when it seems to be very serious and I can't do anything on my own. Otherwise, I treat myself.'

Similarly, Raymonde told of one day experiencing 'pain all over'. She took analgesics but the pain persisted. She then consulted her doctor but:

> The doctor didn't know how to treat me; he gave me anti-inflammatory pain-killers which just relieved the pain a little for a while, that is all. And it still hurt a lot. Then, he did finally send me for some blood test and he found something he didn't understand. Then in the end, after I don't know how long, he sent me to a rheumatologist who found the diagnosis: it was rhizomelic pseudopolyarthritis which he treated with cortisone for 2 years. But the other one, he should have sent me earlier!

Based on this episode, Raymonde thinks that general practitioners 'hold on to patients' and she decided thereafter to go directly to a specialist, believing she is as competent as her GP in assessing the appropriateness of such recourse, when she cannot manage to treat herself.

Thérèse's (a librarian) story also illustrates this phenomenon:

> In 2004, I had terrible diarrhoea. My doctor gave me a treatment that didn't work, he changed the treatment endlessly but he didn't send me for any tests,

no coloscopy or anything. It went on like that for several months. So I tried lots of things like homeopathic remedies but that didn't work either. I lost a lot of weight; but my doctor still did nothing. And then, I had a neighbour who also had diarrhoea; she was treated by the same doctor, and then she died. So I went to hospital and I asked to see a gastroenterologist who did a coloscopy. In fact, there was nothing. But on the other hand, they found that my neighbour had cancer; she went to the hospital too to see a gastroenterologist. It was me who pushed her to go. I told her, 'this diarrhoea is not normal'. And well, she had a tumour that was too big, it was too late! And now she is dead! And as for me, since there were no intestinal problems, they did a scan. They found I had gallstones in the pancreas and diabetes. So, I changed my GP. But that's twice now I have changed, because I was not happy with the first two! So now, I only go for simple things, for which I still need a prescription: infections for example, cystitis, things like that, small, occasional problems. But if I have what I need at home, I don't go, I manage on my own. Otherwise, if I can't solve the problem, I go directly to a specialist.

Because of Thérèse's unfortunate experiences, she now only consults her doctor for small problems ('simple things').

As we can note, the public authorities' recommendation to consult a doctor for serious pathologies and to self-medicate for benign cases is here turned on its head. The patients' accounts are peppered with stories in which they demonstrate their mistrust in the knowledge of doctors and particularly in their capability to identify the seriousness of their problem. Patricia (a salesperson) said she no longer consults doctors to manage the ailments of her daily life and thus justifies her preference for going straight to A and E when her problem is sufficiently serious to not attempt to manage it alone. Equally, Liliane (a 52-year-old graphic designer) explained: 'I don't have a GP. I can manage on my own. If I really need to, when it is an emergency, I call SOS-médecins' (the French emergency medical telephone service).

Some express mistrust towards doctors whose role they believe is reduced to that of a medicine prescriber. This observation challenges the widely held belief that patients always expect their doctor to provide a prescription. However, to the contrary, for Henri (a tax advisor), the doctor's role is precisely to exercise his/her competence in the field of pharmacology. He said: 'One day, I tore a muscle in my thigh, I was doing a lot of sport; I saw a doctor to find out what I should take, and he told me 'it needs rest'. So I don't go anymore! It's a waste of time!'[9] For her part, Julie regrets what consultations are often reduced to: 'If it is just to get medicines, well, there is no point! That's not what we want from doctors!' Similarly, Raymonde complained about the fact that her doctor was happy to just prescribe analgesics, reproaching him for having delayed sending her for the necessary tests and referring her to a rheumatologist capable of making a correct diagnosis. The role of the doctor is thus not necessarily conceived of as that of a medicine prescriber.

An avoidance strategy

In all of these examples, a bad experience has generated a reluctance to return to seeking consultations thought to be pointless, even harmful. The choice of strategy is thus rooted in a desire to avoid the GP, when the subjects fear they may receive poor therapeutic care. A judgement on the limits of their doctor's competence can also encourage subjects to bypass their GP and consult a specialist directly. In this context, self-medication appears either the preferred course of action or a stopgap measure (for lack of direct access to a professional thought to be more competent). While the official recommendations tell the subjects to deal with *benign* or *serious* situations by taking recourse to self-medication or to a GP respectively, we notice that some subjects are more willing to respond either by means of self-medication or by consulting a specialist doctor. Yet, the act of bypassing a GP by going directly to a specialist is today hindered by public policies, notably by the establishment of a 'care pathway' which obliges people to consult a GP who alone can decide on the appropriateness of referring the patient to a specialist colleague. In addition, those who choose to see a specialist without being referred by their GP can face financial sanctions. The high financial cost of a non-prescribed consultation with a specialist (a result of both this financial sanction and the fact that many specialist doctors charge over the standard fee) leads some patients to avoid this strategy, and consequently they either take recourse to self-medication or forego any care at all.

In the case cited above, it is only when her diarrhoea and weight loss became too worrying that Thérèse decided to see a specialist, following a period in which she tried to mitigate her symptoms by ineffective self-medication. Consequently, in some situations, self-medication is not so much a choice but a fallback strategy, for want of a consultation with an authority thought to be more competent than oneself, the aim being to circumvent a doctor.[10] In response to the notion of 'responsibility' invoked in the official documents advocating self-medication and perceived as the 'self-care of certain troubles and afflictions' (Coulomb and Baumelou, 2007: 13), the subjects demonstrate a different 'responsibility' that is tantamount to knowing how to bypass a doctor, or how to assert oneself when faced with a doctor considered incapable. Béatrice, a 36-year-old auditor of public funds, one day experienced an acute toothache which did not go away. She consulted her dentist who 'saw nothing there' and who saw no need to do an x-ray of her teeth, telling her there was nothing abnormal there. The pain persisted. Béatrice then took high doses of analgesics, which only alleviated the pain temporarily. A year and a half later, the pain was still there, sporadically. She ended up consulting another dentist who told her: 'You have a huge cavity, it must date back two or three years; it needs a root canal procedure!' Today Béatrice reproaches herself for having 'given all the power to the first dentist' and for not having 'insisted and persuaded him that this pain needed attention' since she was not able to do it herself – and for having walked away from her responsibilities. The valorisation of responsibility here applies to the activity of the patient taking recourse to a professional in a field not suitable for self-medication since the therapeutic care involves a technical, or surgical, procedure. This responsibilisation does not therefore necessarily imply recourse to self-medication, but it assumes the subject takes an active role in medical care, one form of which is to put pressure on a health professional. The accounts that demonstrate the need to know how to circumvent a doctor thus do not only concern the medicinal management of problems. This is also the case for Ghislaine, an accountant, who had a melanoma. She explained:

> It was of several different colours. I wanted to have it removed for aesthetic reasons. It didn't hurt but it was very unsightly, I had a hang up about it. I consulted a doctor. But he didn't want to touch it. I saw another one but it was the same. It dragged on. Both doctors thought there was no need to intervene and neither of them referred me to a dermatologist. It was only when I showed it to a third one much later on that I was sent to a specialist. He, this specialist, then analysed it and discovered it was malign! Now I don't wait for GPs to send me to specialists anymore; I go myself if I think that it could be serious and that I can't treat it myself.

Exercising one's responsibility here takes a meaning other than choosing one's treatment. For her it meant knowing how to overcome the deficiencies of one professional by a personal action or choice. Therefore, while self-medication entails responsibilisation, responsibilisation does not necessarily entail self-medication.

Criticising medical work cannot be confused with criticising biomedicine. Anthropology has shown that recourse to other (alternative or non-conventional) medicines is partly rooted in a disillusionment with allopathic medicine, with reasons as diverse as the fragmented approach to the body, not taking the patients' discourse seriously enough, or again the adverse side effects of the pharmaceuticals prescribed (*Anthropologie et Santé*, 2011). Yet, as we can see, the users' disillusionment does not necessarily lead them to other types of medicine. It can induce them to want to make their own medicinal choices, potentially linked to divergent etiological or therapeutic schemas, without for all that challenging allopathic medicine itself. By choosing to self-medicate, the subjects do not substitute one type of medicine for another, but one medicinal use for another, or one competence for another. In particular, the subjects can decide to treat themselves because of a different interpretation of the symptom in question (Fainzang, 1997; Sarradon-Eck, 2007). Jean-Pierre suffered from an endless runny nose and sneezing that he interpreted as due to allergies and for which he consulted his doctor. The doctor thought it was just a cold and prescribed drops to prevent rhinitis. But Jean-Pierre was convinced that his affliction was the result of pollution because the episodes stopped when he went on holiday to the sea. So he decided to never go back to see his doctor for that problem, and now takes antihistamines on his own initiative.

However, the avoidance of a medical consultation, which is what self-medication sometimes amounts to, does not always mean the doctor's competence is being challenged. It can be based on a distrust of the medicines that the doctor might prescribe (Britten, 1994, 1996; Chamberlain et al. 2011). The practice of self-medication notably results from the subjects' anxiety as regards certain categories of medicines which leads them to want to manage their treatment themselves. Jocelyne, who suffered from sinusitis, explained: 'I know what he will prescribe if I go to see him – he will give me antibiotics but I don't want them, so I am going to try to sort it out myself.' Gérard suffered from severe back pain: 'Anyway, I can't see what else he will give me apart from anti-inflammatories! But I don't tolerate them. There is nothing else to do but take painkillers! So, there is no point in going to see him for that.' The subjects themselves then have to put in place the modalities of the treatment, taking care not to consume some classes of medicines, contrary to what the doctor would prescribe. It is also to avoid consultations (the costs they entail and the medicinal consumption they induce) that Véronique, a literature teacher, tries out 'consultations' with her friends during which she attempts to identify people's health problems using their 'aura'.

Suspicion of a medicine and fear that taking it may be inappropriate (whether it has been advised by a pharmacist or chosen by herself) is what drives Josiane (a physiotherapist) to resort to radiesthesia in order to check whether the treatment is suitable for her. 'He moves his antenna over the medicines to see if they react in order to test which ones respond,' she explained.

The choice to self-medicate and its modalities therefore refer to practical and symbolic logics. We will see later that these dimensions are also at the base of strategies designed to control the risk associated with self-medication and with medicines, and to maximise the efficacy of the products consumed.

On the whole, the subjects' behaviours as regards medical authority can be organised into two categories:

- One scenario is where the subjects justify their recourse to self-medication by the fact that they think there is no use in seeing a doctor. This is the case for example when, having previously consulted a doctor for a symptom thought to be analogous, they think they already know what should be done. In this case, self-medication consists of trying to reproduce, identically or with some adaptations, a treatment previously prescribed by a doctor, since the subject has acquired (or thinks he/she has acquired) knowledge on the appropriate therapy. It is a model of 'now, I know', where the doctor is assigned a competence and the practice consists of replicating or modifying this.[11] This model includes the subjects who, after having consulted and been prescribed the same treatment as the previous time for similar symptoms, react by saying 'next time, I'll know there is no point going to the doctor' (even if the case is serious), and those who, resistant to taking certain medicines that would certainly be prescribed if they consulted a doctor, prefer to try to resolve their affliction by a different means, based on the knowledge they have about the medicinal alternatives.
- Alternately, the subjects justify their recourse to self-medication by the fact that they believe going to a doctor can be dangerous. This is the case when

self-medication aims, not to reproduce a previous opinion of a doctor who is recognised as competent, but contrarily to escape from what is considered as their incompetence. The very notion of 'delay in diagnosis' (Sand Andersen, 2010), cited by doctors hostile to self-diagnosis in order to emphasis the inherent risks (see chapter 1), is cited and mirrored by the subjects to justify self-medication. Believing the delay to be caused by a doctor who has not been able to see the problem and unsatisfied with his/her expertise (the failure to make a diagnosis or the failure of the treatment proposed), they say they would now rather treat themselves, or 'sort it out on my own', at least when they believe themselves capable. It is a model of 'I know as much as he/she does', or even 'I know better than him/her'. It is therefore the gap left by a disappointing experience or a dissatisfaction with the medical institution that is sometimes filled by self-medication.

What is at stake here is the subject's evaluation of his/her competence in treating the illness *versus* the doctor's. It is worth noting that, not only is the risk of a 'delay in diagnosis' mentioned by the health professionals hostile to self-medication in fact often echoed by the users when they believe that a delay was caused by a doctor who could not 'see' or 'treat' the problem, but also that this mistrust can alternately be held towards a pharmacist: Vera, a 33-year-old architect, had regular stomach pains. On the advice of a colleague who also suffered stomach aches, she took a medicine whose name she had forgotten. But the treatment did not work. Alongside the pain, she suffered from nausea. So she then asked the opinion of a pharmacist who concluded that she had gastroesophageal reflux and proposed an antacid. She followed this treatment but the pains persisted. Finally, she consulted a doctor who referred her for a gastroscopy which revealed the presence of very resistant helicobacter[12] for which the doctor had to prescribe three antibiotic therapies. This episode had led her to mistrust pharmacists who she believes are not competent to analyse pain. She has thus decided to no longer take recourse to the expertise of a pharmacist to whom she attributes a knowledge that is no better than her colleagues'. A harboured distrust of a health professional and his/her medical work because of a negative experience incites subjects to take recourse to someone judged more competent: to a doctor rather than a pharmacist, to a specialist doctor rather than a GP, or even to oneself rather than a pharmacist or doctor.

Sociologists have highlighted the crisis of confidence affecting medicine and its repercussions on the reconfiguration of the social space in healthcare involving a redefinition of professional territories (Aïach *et al.*, 1994; Saliba, 1994; Broclain, 1994), its effect on the relationship the users maintain with the health services (Cresson and Schweyer, 2000), and also on the development of patient associations and the judicialisation of medicine (Rabeharisoa and Callon, 1999; Barbot, 2002; Fillion, 2009). Thus they highlighted the transformations undergone by medical institutions resulting from the erosion of the clinical tradition and developments in biomedicine (Dodier, 2003), and the decline in medical power (Hassenteufel, 1999) heralded by the loss of doctors' power to influence public policy decisions.

However, the object of this distrust is sometimes not so much medicine itself or the medical institution but the people that represent it; and so the institution itself is not necessarily called into question. This applies here since it is most often the judgement on the incompetence of a specific professional that dictates the decision either to take recourse to another, for example a more specialised holder of medical knowledge (although distrust can sometimes be expressed towards specialist doctors too), or to take no recourse to them at all and self-medicate instead. This demonstrates the relevance of Giddens' (1987) distinction between trust in expert systems and trust in people, even though what is at play here is a relative collusion between the two, around the doctor's expertise and professional know-how.

On examining tangible situations studied in the field, it appears that the link between the identification of symptoms and self-medication is forged on four principle models: an empirical model, a moral model, a cognitive model and a substitutive model.

1   An empirical model in which the symptom is familiar (but not necessarily benign), leading the subjects to consider themselves capable of treating it. The identification relies on the experience the subjects have, on which they base their conclusion that a consultation would be useless.

2   A moral model, concerning the register of good behaviour or of moral-social judgement: the symptom relates to a part of the body that the subjects think should be kept hidden or relates to an activity about which the subjects fear the doctor's judgement (for example, sexual activity).

3   A cognitive model: this can involve a symptom not recognised by the doctors, or not identified as pathological by the doctors (Risor, 2010), or indeed a symptom to which the subjects attribute an interpretation which leads them to manage it in their own way, or a symptom that the subjects have acquired personal knowledge about – a knowledge that can be individual and not shared, or collective and transmitted by third parties.

4   A substitutive model: the symptom is not necessarily well known to the subjects but a conviction that the doctor is incapable of managing this symptom leads them to choose to self-medicate, particularly when the symptom has already been experienced, and has already been the reason for a previous consultation during which the patients believe they did not receive a satisfactory response from the doctor.

Part of the reason for choosing to self-medicate is therefore based on a logic of expertise, resulting from a judgement of competence – notably from a judgement on what the subjects consider to be incompetence *of* doctors or of *their* doctor. Some attribute this failure to the overly generalised knowledge of GPs or express their doubts about whether the GPs are really disposed to referring their patients to specialist colleagues, while others apply this judgement to a particular doctor (often their GP).[13] In these conditions, the choice to self-medicate is rooted in the desire to avoid a medical consultation or is anchored in the failures of medical work.

Such an analysis diverges from that of Hammer (2010) who showed that lay criticisms are almost never expressed as a challenge to professional competence, and relate less to doctors and their qualities than to the institutional context (hierarchy, bureaucracy) in which they practice. It also differs from Gagnon's (1998) analysis that the principle of autonomy has allowed patients, ultimately, to challenge the superiority of medical norms over individual norms in the assessment of the illness and the therapy. It is not necessarily the medical norms themselves that are questioned; it can simply be, as we have seen, a questioning of the competences of individual doctors in enacting these norms. Finally, while the subjects' self-medication corresponds to a *rupture in dependence* on medical authority – or even, as an affirmation of their autonomy, to a *challenge* of medical authority (Gagnon, 1998) – it sometimes corresponds more to a challenge of the competence of this authority.

Notes

1 The title of this chapter is an homage to Marshall Sahlins' important book, *Culture and Practical Reason* (1976), where he simultaneously considered both the practical and symbolic dimensions of the study of societies.
2 What is new in France is that it is now actively encouraged by the public authorities.
3 We should add to this the role played by religious cultural origin (cf. Fainzang, 2001b, 2005), as a greater valorisation of self-medication can be observed amongst people of Protestant origins than among other groups in the French population.
4 A dimension also found in very different socio-cultural contexts (cf. for example Baxerres (2010) on the uses of industrial medicines in Benin).
5 If a doctor charges more than the standard fee, the patient is eligible to pay for the excess since their medical insurance only refunds the standard fee.
6 Even if the doctors continue to be against it for the stated reason that it could cause a delay in diagnosis and give rise to incorrect medicinal use. We will return to this point in Chapter 5.
7 The troubles most frequently mentioned were colds, coughs, fevers, stomach pains, digestive problems, back pains and insomnia.
8 In fact she takes a hypnotic, which was 'advised' to her by her pharmacist for her sleeping troubles.
9 In this regard, we can appreciate the difficulties contained in the French National Health Authority's decision to promote non-medicinal prescriptions (cf. Progress report on the 'Development of the prescription of validated non-medicinal therapies': www.has-sante.fr/portail/jcms/c_1059795/developpement-de-la-prescription-de-therapeutiques-non-medicamenteuses-validees).
10 Strategies to avoid a specialist doctor with whom the subject is not satisfied also exist, although more rarely, giving rise to, here again, either self-medication or another consultation with a different doctor. The subject can however then fear being reproached for 'medical nomadism'.
11 Even though self-medication is also nourished by other sources of knowledge, as we will see further on.
12 A bacteria that infects the mucous membrane of the human stomach wall.
13 Which they do not dare (or do not know how) to change.

References

Aïach P. and Cèbe D., 1991, *Expression des symptômes et conduites de maladie*, Paris: Editions de l'Inserm/Doin.

Aïach P., Fassin D. and Saliba, J., 1994, 'Crise, pouvoir et légitimité', in P. Aïach and D. Fassin (eds), *Les métiers de la santé, enjeux de pouvoir et quête de légitimité*, Paris: Anthropos-Economica, 9–42.

Anthropologie et Santé, 2011, 2, 'Anthropologie des soins non conventionnels du cancer' [http://anthropologiesante.revues.org/147].

Barbot J., 2002, *Les malades en mouvements. La médecine et la science à l'épreuve du sida*, Paris: Balland.

Barthe J.F., 1990, 'Connaissance profane des symptômes et recours thérapeutiques', *Revue française de sociologie*, XXXI, 2 : 283–296.

Baxerres C., 2010, *Du médicament informel au médicament libéralisé. Les offres et les usages du médicament pharmaceutique industriel à Cotonou (Bénin)*, thèse EHESS/ Université Abomey-Calavi.

Blenkinsopp A. and Bradley C., 1996, 'Patients, society and the increase of self-medication', *BMJ*, 312: 629–632.

Britten N., 1994, 'Patients' ideas about medicines. A qualitative study in a general practice population', *British Journal of General Practice*, 44: 465–468.

Britten N., 1996, 'Lay views of drugs and medicines: orthodox and unorthodox accounts', in: S.J. Williams, and M. Calnan (eds), *Modern medicine. Lay perspectives and experiences*, London: UCL Press.

Broclain D., 1994, 'La médecine générale en crise?' in: P. Aïach and D. Fassin (eds), *Les métiers de la santé. Enjeux de pouvoir et quête de légitimité*, Paris: Anthropos, 122–160.

Brodwin P.E., 1994, 'Symptoms and social performances: the case of Diane Reden', in: M.-J. DelVecchio Good, P.E. Brodwin, B.J. Good and A. Kleinman (eds), *Pain as human experience. An anthropological perspective*, Berkeley: University of California Press, 77–99.

Buclin T. and Ammon C. (eds), 2001, *L'automédication: pratique banale, motifs complexes*, Genève: Médecine et Hygiène, Cahiers Médico-Sociaux, 11–29.

Burnier M. and Schneider M.P., 2001, 'De l'automédication à la non-observance thérapeutique', in: T. Buclin and Ammon C. (eds), *L'automédication: pratique banale, motifs complexes*, Genève: Médecine et Hygiène, Cahiers Médico-Sociaux, 89–97.

Burnier M.J. and Jeanneret O., 2001, 'L'automédication, une pratique en quête de sens: sa place dans le self care et la promotion de la santé', in: T. Buclin and C. Ammon (eds), *L'automédication: pratique banale, motifs complexes*, Genève: Médecine et Hygiène, Cahiers Médico-Sociaux, 11–29.

Chamberlain K., Madden H., Gabe J., Dew K. and Norris P., 2011, Forms of resistance to medications within New Zealand households, *Medische Antropologie*, 23, 2, 299–308.

Collin J., 2007b, 'Du silence des organes au souci de soi: médicament et reconfiguration de la notion de prévention', in: I. Rossi (ed.), *Prévoir et prévoir la maladie. De la divination au pronostic*, Monts: Aux lieux d'être, 139–151.

Collin J., Otero M. and Monnais L., 2006, 'Le médicament entre science, norme et culture', in: J. Collin, M. Otero and L. Monnais (eds), *Le médicament au coeur de la socialité contemporaine. Regards croisés sur un objet complexe*, Montréal: Presses de l'université du Québec, 1–15.

Coulomb A. and Baumelou A., 2007, 'Situation de l'automédication en France et perspectives d'évolution : marché, comportements, positions des acteurs', Rapport établi à la demande du ministère de la santé et de la protection sociale, 32 p.

Cresson G. and Schweyer F.-X. (eds), 2000, *Les usagers du système de soins*, Rennes: Les Editions de l'ENSP.

DelVecchio Good M.J., Brodwin P.E., Good B.J. and Kleinman A., (eds), 1994, *Pain as human experience. An anthropological perspective*, Berkeley: University of California Press.

DGS/CSA-TMO santé, 2002, *Enquête sur l'automédication*, October.

Dodier N., 2003, *Leçons politiques de l'épidémie de sida*, Paris: Ed. de l'EHESS.

Fainzang S., 1997, 'Les stratégies paradoxales. Réflexions sur la question de l'incohérence des conduites de malades', *Sciences Sociales et Santé*, 15, 3: 5–23.

Fainzang S., 2001b, *Médicaments et société. Le patient, le médecin et l'ordonnance*, Paris: Presses Universitaires de France.

Fainzang S., 2005, 'Religious attitudes toward prescriptions, medicines and doctors in France', *Culture, Medicine and Psychiatry*, 29, 4: 457–476.

Fillion E., 2009, *A l'épreuve du sang contaminé*. Paris: Ed. de l'EHESS.

Gagnon E., 1998, 'L'avènement médical du sujet. Les avatars de l'autonomie en santé', *Sciences sociales et santé*, 16, 1: 49–74.

Giddens A., 1987, *La constitution de la société*, Paris: PUF.

Good B.J. and M.-J. Delvecchio-Good, 1981, 'The meaning of symptoms: a cultural hermeneutic model for clinical practice', in: L. Eisenberg and A. Kleinman (eds), *The relevance of social science for medicine*, Dordrecht/Boston/Lancaster: D. Reidel Publishing Company, 165–196.

Hammer R., 2010, *Expériences ordinaires de la médecine. Confiances, croyances et critiques profanes*, Zurich/Genève: Ed. Seismo.

Hassenteufel P., 1999, 'Vers le déclin du 'pouvoir médical'?', *Pouvoirs*, 89 : 51–64.

Karsenty S., 1994, 'L'enfant, sa famille et les médicaments: approche sociologique et anthropologique', in: *L'enfant, sa famille et les médicaments*, Paris, Institut de l'Enfance et de la Famille, 4–49.

Karsenty S., 2009, 'Le retour hétéro-déterminé de l'automédication', *Sociologie santé*, 30: 101–117.

Laure P., 1998, 'Enquête sur les usagers de l'automédication: de la maladie à la performance', *Thérapie*, 53, 2: 127–135.

Le Moigne Ph., 1999, *Anxiolytiques, hypnotiques. Les facteurs sociaux de la consommation*. Document of the GDR 'Psychotropes, Politique et Société', 1.

Lecomte T., 1994, 'La consommation pharmaceutique des enfants de moins de 10 ans d'après les données de l'enquête sur la santé et les soins médicaux réalisée en 1991–92', in: *L'enfant, sa famille et les médicaments*, Paris: Institut de l'Enfance et de la Famille, 55–68.

Lecomte T., 1988, 'L'automédication a-t-elle un avenir en 'rance', *Prospective et Santé*, 47–48: 187–190.

McKinlay J., 1975, 'The help seeking behavior of the poor', in: J. Kosa and I. Zola (eds), *Poverty and health: a sociological analysis*, Cambridge, MA: Harvard University Press.

Molina N., 1988, *L'automédication*, Paris: PUF (Coll: Les champs de la santé).

Nichter M. and Vuckovic N., 1994, 'Agenda for an anthropology of pharmaceutical practice', *Social Science and Medicine*, 39, 11: 1509–1525.

Nouguez E., 2007, 'Copies conformes, comportements conformes? Les patients français face au choix des médicaments génériques', *Sociologie santé*, 26 ('Système de santé et discours profanes'), 247–261.

Ostermann G., 1999, 'Aspects psychologiques de l'automédication', in: P. Queneau (ed.), *Automédication, autoprescription, autoconsommation*. Paris: John Libbey, 33–38.

Queneau P., 1999, 'Automédication en antalgiques', in: P. Queneau (ed.), *Automédication, autoprescription, autoconsommation*, Paris : John Libbey, 84–95.

Queneau P., Froudarakis M., Salvador M, Villani P. and Vital-Durand D., 2004, 'Automédication concernant les antalgiques', in: P. Queneau and G. Ostermann (eds), *Le médecin, le malade et la douleur*. Paris: Masson, 389–398.

Rabeharisoa V. and Callon, M., 1999, *Le pouvoir des malades. L'Association française contre les myopathies et la Recherche*. Paris: Presses de l'Ecole des mines.

Raynaud D., 2008, 'Les déterminants du recours à l'automédication', *Revue Française des Affaires Sociales*, 1: 81–94.

Risor M.B., 2010, 'Healing and recovery as a social process among patients with medically unexplained symptoms (MUS)', in: S. Fainzang, H.E. Hem and M.B. Risor (eds), *The taste for knowledge: medical anthropology facing medical realities*, Copenhagen: Aarhus University Press, 133–149.

Sahlins M., 1976, *Culture and practical reason*, Chicago: University of Chicago Press.

Saliba J., 1994, 'Les paradigmes des professions de santé', in: P. Aïach and D. Fassin (eds), *Les métiers de la santé. Enjeux de pouvoir et quête de légitimité*, Paris: Anthropos, 43–85.

Sand Andersen R., 2010, 'Anthropological perspectives on the biomedically defined problem of "patient delay"', in: S. Fainzang, H.E. Hem and M.B. Risor (eds), *The taste for knowledge: medical anthropology facing medical realities*, Copenhagen: Aarhus University Press, 57–68.

Sarradon-Eck A., 2007, 'Le sens de l'observance. Ethnographie des pratiques médicamenteuses de personnes hypertendues', *Sciences sociales et santé*, 25, 2: 5–36.

Sarradon-Eck A., Blanc M.A. and Faure M., 2007, 'Des usagers sceptiques face aux médicaments génériques: une approche anthropologique', *Revue d'épidémiologie et de santé publique*, 55: 179–185.

Saubadu S., 1988, *Enquête sur l'automédication: comparaison de deux groupes*, Thèse Université Paris V.

Steudler F., 1999, 'Aspects sociologiques de l'automédication', in: P. Queneau (ed.), *Automédication, autoprescription, autoconsommation*. Paris, John Libbey, 23–32.

Thoër C., Pierret J. and Lévy J.J., 2008, 'Quelques réflexions sur des pratiques d'utilisation des médicaments hors cadre médical', *Drogues, santé et société*, 7, 1: 19–54.

4   Knowledge and competence

One of the terms of the debate that rages about self-medication is the *competence* (Hunter, 2010) of the users, or rather what the health professionals believe to be their incompetence, which mirrors the distrust subjects sometimes feel towards their doctor. Here, I do not seek to takes sides in this debate. Within the remit of such a study, an anthropologist's role is not to support those who loudly proclaim the existence of a 'lay' knowledge that rivals a professional or 'expert' knowledge,[1] rendering users capable of self-medicating, nor is it to support those who contest this knowledge or who at least reject the competence it would provide in treating oneself through self-medication. Because it is indeed this issue of knowledge that is raised alongside that of competence. Studies into the meaning assigned to the practice of self-medication tend to avoid reflecting on the relationship to knowledge it implies. The authors of the CSA/CECOP (2007) study identified three groups of patients: those for whom self-medication means 'treating oneself without going to see a doctor', those for whom it is 'seeing a pharmacist to treat oneself without seeing a doctor', and those who think it is 'choosing medicines oneself with which to treat oneself'. Yet, these three categories do not hold the same status as regards the relationship with medical power, and especially not in terms of the knowledge it is based on, since the first phrase emphasises lay knowledge as opposed to professional knowledge, the second emphasises pharmacist knowledge as opposed to that of the doctor, while the third only emphasises the user's role as a 'consumer'. The posture of the user towards knowledge remains unexplored even though these categories can overlap as regards this issue.

We have seen that self-medication is the object of some reservations, notably from the doctors, because they consider it to be often dangerous for the very reason that it is based on insufficient knowledge. They invoke the risk involved either of a 'delay in diagnosis' or of an incorrect medicinal use. Inversely, recourse to self-medication for the subjects is an expression of their claim to competence, based on their knowledge. I will examine how the diverse forms of knowledge mobilised in self-medication are constituted in order to define the stakes involved in the assertion or denial of this competence. When broaching the matter of user knowledge, it is customary to oppose so-called lay knowledge with professional or expert knowledge. Freidson (1984) proposed the concept of a lay system of reference to account for what leads individuals to share information about their health problems and the agents capable of treating them to guide their choices of care-providers or health services. However we should note that a lay system of reference for Freidson is equivalent to a hierarchical process of searching for information that begins with the least informed and experienced and finishes with those who have the most information and experience, before arriving at the medical care system itself (Aïach and Cèbe, 1991: 12), whereas, as this material shows, sometimes the opposite occurs: deception with the medical system leads the subjects to turn to 'lay consultants' who are, for example, members of their close family or friends. Social scientists then started to use this distinction to account for the difference between the expert knowledge of health professionals and the 'lay' knowledge of ill people. The notion of 'lay knowledge' coupled with that of the 'expert patient' has been validated by numerous works and numerous observers in the field of health. They believe that citizens are equipped with their own resources, knowledge and competence. Some saw illness as an 'autodidact' episode (Jouet et al., 2010: 69), others advocated for institutional recognition of illness experience (Tourette-Turgis, 2010); still others underlined the limitations associated with patient knowledge and the paradox it contains, since knowledge simultaneously involves growing uncertainty and is conscious of its limits (Topçu et al., 2008).

Anthropologists however object to using the notion of 'lay' knowledge, not because this would deny the specificity of professional knowledge but because the notion implies taking the point of view of the experts – here, medical experts – and consists of defining this knowledge in opposition to that of the doctors, in other words defining it by *what it is not*, as *non*-specialised or *non*-acquainted with medical science. It thus consists of perceiving things through the eyes and the judgement of the doctor, a perspective contrary to the anthropologists' decision to not assume or endorse the medical perspective, but rather to study an object starting from the thought categories of the people studied. Good (1998) thus denounced the use of the concept of 'lay' which would signify establishing a relationship of domination between medical knowledge and popular knowledge.

Here I will not refer to the opposition between 'lay' knowledge and 'professional' knowledge, not only because the use of these notions implies adopting a medical perspective, or because it involves ranking them (Good *et al.*, 1998), or even because this distinction pertains to the idea that the differences in contents involve categorical differences between patients and health professionals (Balcou-Debussche, 2006), but also because, on one hand, the distinction does not hold in the context of self-medication since it is the subject who provides the expertise and becomes the expert in managing the affliction, and, on the other hand, because, in this context, these categories overlap substantially.

For their part, Akrich *et al.* (2010) rightly highlighted the difficulty of finding a perfect clarification of the notion of lay despite the abundance of literature that exists on the subject. Upon reading the texts involved in the controversy in environmental health for example, these authors proposed two types of distinction: firstly, one that separates 'lay expertise' and experience-based knowledge, and secondly, one that differentiates this experience-based knowledge from professional knowledge. Lay expertise refers to the ability that non-specialists can have to appropriate scientific knowledge, understand the debates running through the research community and use some publications and academic data for their own purposes (p. 26). The notion of 'experience-based knowledge' or 'experience-based expertise' however relates to a type of knowledge that is radically different to professional knowledge and the result of singular experience.

However, this division implies a lay knowledge that partners professional knowledge (lay expertise) and another type of lay knowledge that ruptures with it (experience-based knowledge). This division, in turn, raises a difficulty in that it maintains a radical opposition between the lay system and the expert system. Yet, I will show that not only can these categories interpenetrate but that the very sources of knowledge from which they are nourished do not have defined nor watertight boundaries.

Between experience and information

The practice of self-medication raises the question of the means by which users acquire knowledge about the drugs they consume. User competence, affirmed by some and rejected by others, is linked to an affirmation of a knowledge relating to two orders of reality. One is acquired by experience, the other by information.

Between experience and knowledge

In reference to illness, the notion of experience contains two acceptations: it relates to both *the fact of feeling* (experiencing) something (a sensation, symptoms) and to *the fact of knowing this thing* by having already felt (experienced) it. Knowledge is a potentiality specific to this experience, to the point that it confers a form of authority to the person having had the experience. When subjects take recourse to self-medication in reaction to symptoms already experienced, they believe that they can deal with these symptoms because they *know* them. The link established here between experience and knowledge is the basis of the process of acquiring a competence.[2] In some patient associations, the recognition of knowledge based on experience is the foundation of their practice of offering members the support of other patients suffering from the same ailment as them. This is the case for example in former alcoholics' associations, the prominent forefathers of contemporary patient associations, whose doctrine is that caring for somebody suffering from alcoholism can only be done among peers: it is necessary to have experienced the illness oneself, and thus know it, to be able to manage the care of another. The members of the associations are credited with knowledge as a direct result of their intimate experience of the illness (cf. Fainzang, 1996). It is the experience that confers a competence.

The choice of medicines is of course also linked to parameters other than knowledge. It is partly derived from the galenic aspect or from the organoleptic[3] quality of the medicine. Akrich (1995) highlighted the degree to which the presentation of the drug – its packaging, conditioning, instructions and galenic formulation – influences the way it is used and the meaning it is ascribed. In this regard, while the galenic formulation is a key factor in ensuring observance of prescribed treatments (Guerci *et al.*, 2002),[4] it is also an important aspect in the context of self-medication. Thus, the subjects sometimes adapt a former prescription by substituting one medicine for another when the taste or the way it must be taken do not suit them: some for example swap a suppository prescription for their 'equivalent' in pill or ointment form; others look for a substitute to a formerly prescribed pill because they do not like its bitterness; others again choose to buy the medicines they prefer directly. The reason for such a preference varies: comfort in taking the drug, a judgement on the risk or, inversely, on the efficacy of a medicine. Starkly contrasting attitudes were noted concerning for example the intake of bitter medicines. Some rejected such products because of their unpleasant taste (this is the case for those who prefer film-coated tablets); some, in contrast, preferred these products thinking it is preferable for a medicine to taste bad so it does not become a consumer product like any other (Gérard thus disapproved of the sweet, pleasant taste of syrups for children: 'They want to turn them into drug addicts! They complain that people take too many medicines but they shouldn't give children a taste for it when they are very little!'), while others associate the unpleasant taste of a medicine with an increased efficacy. However, the covert information contained in the galenic aspect of a medicine is never the only factor. It comes in addition to the other information the users obtain which serves to build and consolidate the knowledge they acquire on the subject.

The modalities of medicinal use often result from knowledge acquired from the subjects' personal history and their experience of the ailment but also from knowledge of the effects felt in the past following the intake of a certain substance. Thus when medicines are taken in situations that differ from those in which they are normally prescribed, this use, which is called 'misuse' or deliberate 'change of use', is in itself an expression of knowledge, acquired through experience, on the effect that the given substance can produce.[5]

The subjects' knowledge is fed by several different sources for the same affliction. Built gradually, the knowledge acquired can lead them to refuse prescribed medicines and choose to manage the ailment by another means, on their own initiative. We can recall Denise's case; she refused to take antibiotics prescribed by her doctor to treat her sore throat because she thought he prescribed them too often without this solving the problem since the pharyngitis kept coming back. She then tried to treat herself, alone, with homeopathic medicines but when her sore throat persisted, and having learnt from a friend that the pains could be the result of sugar intolerance, she then chose to undertake an 'experiment' to test this hypothesis. This she judged to be conclusive and so was reassured in her decision to no longer take antibiotics to solve the problem.

Knowledge concerning a medicine is built on a conviction as to its efficacy, via the establishment of what constitutes proof. In Denise's case, it is an empirical failure (the failure of the antibiotic treatment) which leads to a conceptual rupture, for which she seeks coherence in her personal history. The medicinal management of her ailment is based on a thought system that mixes medical logic with idiosyncratic categories. What this proof is based on of course differs depending on the health system in question (Naraindas, 2006). In the context of self-medication, there is no system to which a population collectively adheres since it is based on individual mechanisms – that follow personal criteria – of how the proof is demonstrated or administrated. The proof is established by means of idiosyncratic ingredients since the subjects construct a personal discourse on the etiology of their affliction and on the efficacy of their treatments but also borrow from medical discourse, in producing a causality based for example on a logic of 'allergy', or in trying to verify or test a hypothesis, a diagnosis or a medicine with experimentation. Of course, the test is not double-blind and the experiment does not meet scientific criteria, but it remains, for the subjects, a decisive element in the evaluation and the construction of their knowledge, whether relating to medicines or other substances, the effects of which are experienced in their bodies.

On this point, Jason Corburn (cited in Akrich *et al.*, 2010) made a distinction between lay knowledge and professional knowledge based on the means by which it is acquired: one is acquired by experience, the other by experiment. However, although it is true that the opposition between experience and experiment draws a boundary between these two types of knowledge, crediting the latter type with a scientific status,[6] we should note on the other hand the difficulty the users of self-medication have in making such a distinction, in that they sometimes undertake what they consider to be an experiment – although one that does not follow scientific rules – in order to validate their conviction concerning the origin of a symptom,[7] or the efficacy or the safety of a remedy.

The knowledge individuals gather about medicines also comes from advice from people they interact with, who may be close to them or not (family, friends, colleagues, neighbours, association members or networks), to the point that other people's experiences are liable to become substitutes for personal experience. Indeed, it is not rare for subjects to say they are not familiar with the medicine they have decided to take but have 'heard about it' from someone who is. It was because Christiane was advised a hypnotic that her mother uses regularly and consequently has experience of that she decided to take it to resolve her sleeping problems. However, the impact of the information or advice provided by an acquaintance is extremely variable considering the degree to which the subject credits this person's opinion, which depends on his/her place in the kinship network and on the relationship the subject has with him/her. Ultimately, what is sometimes confusingly called 'experience' is not always one's own but also that of others.

Knowledge and information

Alongside knowledge acquired through experience, we can find knowledge acquired through information, gleaned from diverse sources, allowing the users to appropriate part of the specialists' knowledge. An examination of the empirical situations in which subjects practice self-medication shows that they never confront the symptom and the choice to take one medicine or another alone. They receive information from different sources as varied as health campaigns, previous medical consultations, pharmacists, family and friends, pharmaceutical leaflets and the media – notably the press, television and Internet (Akrich and Méadel, 2004; Fox, Ward and O'Rourke, 2005).

Information about medicines is partly provided by doctors, especially within the framework of previous prescriptions (Karsenty, 1994, 2009). The knowledge diffused is then appropriated, even if the subjects may subsequently reinterpret it. Liliane (a 52-year-old graphic designer) treats her son's laryngitis with Celestene (a corticoid with a powerful anti-inflammatory action) ever since a doctor prescribed it to him when he had the same affliction at 18 months old. Now, she gives it to him on her own initiative, thinking she knows what to do 'as soon as he feels a bit breathless'. The knowledge of this medicine and what she thinks she knows about its use had thus been transmitted directly from the doctor. Equally, it is because his doctor had interpreted his stomach pains to be the result of stress that Richard now turns to self-medication as soon as he gets a stomach ache (for which he takes tranquilisers), thinking he now knows this pain and that there is no longer any need to consult a doctor when it reoccurs. Knowledge of a medicine chosen for self-medication when a given symptom appears is transmitted both by the information gained from a previous experience of the affliction and by the way in which it was managed by a professional. 'Lay' knowledge and the behaviours it brings about – which are often condemned by health professionals (Katz, 1984) – thus appear to often be the unexpected result of patients assimilating the discourses and knowledge transmitted by the medical milieu.

Information originating in medical discourse, which constitutes a part of the 'knowledge' the subjects build up about the medicines, is also transmitted through the messages of public health campaigns. But this information is often partial to the extent that we can question the type of knowledge it actually permits. Here we can use the example of the high consumption of antibiotics in France for which the consequences are not simply economic but also therapeutic, considering the resistance this overconsumption causes and the poor prospect of finding molecules able to replace the current antibiotics in the near future. The issue of diffusing knowledge about drugs is a concern for both health professionals and public authorities to such an extent that an entire branch of public health has developed based on what is referred to as 'patient education'. Recognition of the problem posed by the overconsumption of antibiotics induced the French National Health Insurance Fund to produce an information clip in 2006 aimed at the general public. This clip was a key part of the information campaign that used the watchword, 'Antibiotics are not automatic'. The explicit message was that antibiotics should not be consumed excessively and that a prescription of these drugs should not be sought at all costs.[8] However, incomplete information leads to the creation of false knowledge and has the effect of promoting behaviours contrary to those sought. We can note that, in order to conform to the injunction contained in this message, some patients, firmly believing such overconsumption is harmful and claiming to be perfectly aware of the fact that it is dangerous to take too many antibiotics, claim that when they do consume them, they take care to stop the treatment as soon as the symptoms disappear which often means from the second or third day of the treatment. Their adherence to a badly understood but also badly transmitted message leads them to the opposite result to that desired since they do not take the drugs correctly, or we could say that here, they do not take them enough,[9] thereby accentuating the risk of resistance. We can measure here the risks inherent in information campaigns overly focussed on imparting a behavioural norm without actually providing genuine information. In this case, these patients act against a medical norm by seeking to conform to it. When not coupled with the transmission of genuine knowledge, the diffusion of a norm can lead to the production of a deviance.

The knowledge the users possess about medicines also partly comes from information diffused by the pharmaceutical industry, through pharmaceutical leaflets. Regarding these leaflets, Akrich (1995) noted that they 'partly extend the medical consultation and the interaction with the pharmacist by explicitly offering a definition of the medicine and its uses' (p. 132). In fact, they can not necessarily *extend* it but potentially *replace* it, when no consultation is sought (and this is the case for self-medication) and the subjects try to find in the leaflet both a description of their symptoms and the therapy necessary for the ailment to which the symptoms correspond. By reading a pharmaceutical leaflet, the subjects gather advice: they compare the indications with the symptoms to be managed in order to make a diagnosis and give themselves a self-prescription – or in order to decide on a use for a family member, especially a child (Jonville and Autret, 1994). The leaflets sometimes cruelly lack information, whether about the indications or the posology, stating that one should refer to a medical prescription. When the drug indications are deliberately omitted, Madeleine Akrich remarked, 'it is difficult not to see this as a restriction on patient rights in the name of both the competence which is conferred by the position of specialist and of what is considered to be a diminishment of the person being treated, because of his/her pathology' (1995: 136). However, subjects can choose to resist this model, basing their actions on information mined elsewhere (for example on the Internet or from people around them) or previously (in the case of a previous prescription) or, as we have seen, based on their own experience. Beyond the power relationship, what is at play here is very much a relationship to knowledge. The leaflet can provide information to patients that is liable to make them reluctant to take the treatment because of the indications and side effects detailed. In the context of self-medication, the information provided by these leaflets will guide a large part of the practices and form the basis of a part of the knowledge that the subjects possess on the drugs, to such a point that it is sometimes the accidental reading of a leaflet that leads the user discover that this product could be used to mitigate symptoms he/she sometimes experiences, as illustrated by the case of Françoise discovering the indication of a medicine she had in her domestic pharmacy.

The growing use of the Internet has been the object of numerous studies (Hardey, 2004; Akrich and Méadel, 2004). Patient recourse to medical sites, forums and discussion lists has now become the emblem of the democratisation of knowledge. Following Giddens (1991), Thoer *et al.* (2008) emphasised that the diffusion of health-related information on the Internet allows lay people to 'reappropriate' knowledge and expertise. They showed that some authors (such as Hardey, 2001) 'adopt an optimistic vision of the internet, claiming that this tool contributes to liberating the patient from biomedical domination because it democratises access to knowledge, allows the development of an individual and collective expertise which is based above all on experiential knowledge, different from that of clinicians, and drives alternative modalities of care which promote the empowerment of individuals as regards their health' (Thoër *et al.* 2008: 39).

Evidently, the information gathered on the Internet does not only come from professional sites. It assembles that provided by specialists on websites for the general public, validated or not by health institutions, and that transmitted through the experience of other web users, recounted on the discussion forums – and the two are sometimes mixed in the subjects' accounts. In this regard, through their promotion of the diffusion of knowledge, the patient associations[10] played a pioneering role: within the limited field of an association, this was the precursor to the information sharing between ill people that now takes place on associative sites and forums.

To refine their knowledge on a pathology or a medicine, the subjects also search for information on the Internet when confronted with an unfamiliar symptom. They look for opinions on discussion forums to help them identify the etiology or the seriousness of a symptom (Mechanic, 1980; Garro, 2000). An example of this is provided by Mrs F, mentioned above, who one day experienced a very disagreeable sensation when eating and drinking: a bitter taste filled her mouth whenever she consumed anything. She asked a pharmacist what this could mean but he answered that he didn't know what it could be and that it was not important. The sensation was so unpleasant that she wondered whether there was nevertheless something pathological about it. She considered trying to take antihistamines to manage what she thought could be an allergy. With the bitter taste still bothering her, she went to the discussion forums on the Internet where she discovered that many other people had already experienced this disagreeable sensation and, based on several personal accounts, she learnt that it was caused by the consumption of pine nuts from China[11] – the exact type of nut she had eaten the day before – and that the symptom generally disappears on its own accord after about a week.[12] From then on Mrs F possessed knowledge about this 'symptom' which on one hand reassured her and on the other taught her how to prevent it in the future by not eating the substance that caused the problem, without having had to resort to a medicinal treatment. My own research on this subject led me to discover the testimony of a doctor, on this same forum:

> I am a doctor and this evening my husband told me he has had a bitter taste in his mouth since last night, and so do I! In fact both of us ate some pine nuts last night, which our children didn't and they are not suffering from any taste problems (dysgeusia). Thanks to this forum! While I knew about taste problems linked to medicines (we are not taking any), I didn't know anything about pine nuts!

This reveals that consulting these forums and the 'lay' accounts they contain can also prove a source of information for health professionals.

The media, and the Internet in particular, is thus a powerful vector of information. However, the impact of these diverse sources is not identical for all users, no more than their perceptions of the sources are. Although he is a specialist in computing, Patrick, 32 years old, is very circumspect towards the information diffused on the Web. He is reluctant to search the Internet for medical information, considering that:

> We can never be sure of a website because, even if it is a good one, someone could have put something up there. I have more trust in a book or a magazine because it can't be modified. A book doesn't change! A website is not the same; we can say that it is right but someone could have changed it; it could have been hacked, so it is not trustworthy! It's dangerous!

On the other hand, he is very open to drug advertising which he considers to be authentic, verified information ('A drug advert is trustworthy because there are censorship committees, it is controlled. They can't say anything they like. So it is correct.'). And so he bases his self-medicinal choices on advertising messages. The issue of the reliability of the information received is complex. According to a WHIST study by Inserm (Renahy *et al.*, 2007), 42% of French web users from the general public verify the origin of the information they obtain on the Internet. My own observations have shown that the information is assessed in diverse ways, depending on the individuals and their histories, and on the medium. In contrast to the computer specialist quoted above, Mr L believes the television is more reliable than a magazine because it has a greater number of viewers than a magazine has readers.[13] Self-medication is thus fed by information received from different sources. But the source itself of this knowledge is likely to influence medicinal use. The rationality of such behaviours is of course questionable, in particular when we note the discrepancy that can exist between the sources of information used and the credibility assigned to them.[14]

The subjects consult the Internet because they want to gather a plurality of points of view. Doctors generally take a very dim view of patients referring to the Web in this way. This is sometimes a legitimate concern since some patients are incapable of critically assessing the information gathered, which is often judged to be harmful or false. In this regard, Hardey (2004) explained the dangers of the Internet where the contents are often not differentiated in the eyes of the users. He showed that its architecture allows one to go from an informative space to a commercial one in one simple click. We can agree however that the risk of not always knowing how to discriminate between informative discourse and commercial discourse also exists for the doctor confronted with massive amounts of marketing communications from the pharmaceutical industry. Moreover, according to Romeyer (2008), who analysed the uses of health information on the Internet: 'Contrary to professional fears, the web user appears to distinguish between these two types of information' (p. 31) and the users 'appear to have understood the difference between professional, specialised and scientific medical information distributed by the medical body, and health information from the general public' (p. 40).

In fact, Internet searches are not always carried out in an uncontrolled and erratic way. The patients are sometimes aware of the reliability of some sites and the non-credibility of others. It is not uncommon for patients to assess the information gathered in terms of the medium it appears on even though in some cases the patient's attribution of quality to a source can be rather questionable.[15] For the moment, taking recourse to the Internet is still partly experienced by some patients as an act of transgression; they do so with the feeling of contravening a prohibition and so hide their Internet searches from their doctors. On this point, the major role played by the Internet in transforming medical knowledge and the relationships each person has with information has been well demonstrated by Hardey (2004). He showed that the Internet does not simply produce more thoughtful patients who do not place all their trust in conventional sources of authority, but that it also allows them to question or challenge the opinions of health professionals. As Blech (2005) wrote: 'The Internet weakens the power of doctors and enriches the knowledge of patients'. It is however appropriate to temper such optimism on the subject by referring to the observations of Wyatt *et al.* (2004), doubtless more realistic, that show that the figure of the active, autonomous patient capable of critically assessing information is in fact marginal. According to them, presently, the Internet only amplifies the means of action and reflection of those who already take a critical stance towards the dominant medical doctrines – and, we could add, the medical institution. While, as various works on the subject show, Internet consultations are more often undertaken by people with a certain level of education, or by those used to using information through their professional activities, or as a result of their generational belonging, it does not appear on the other hand that, contrary to Renahy's (2008) claims, health sites on the Internet are only consulted in order to obtain information to complement a medical consultation.

Forums have a particular status in that they, in turn, drive the experience of others. From this point of view, 'recourse to the Internet' cannot be considered in a comprehensive way since it combines recourse to specialist opinions with recourse to 'lay' opinions. The phrase 'consulting the Internet' covers heterogeneous practices since consulting a forum and consulting a professional site are undeniably different social practices. Internet consultations answer to a desire to compare diverse points of view, in other words to draw on academic or professional knowledge *and* experience-based knowledge (one's own and that of others). Where gathering information on the Internet is to combine and compare different registers of knowledge, in return, transmitting one's experience-based knowledge on the Internet is to validate, even officialise, its contents.

Therefore the subjects have several objectives for consulting the Internet: one is to increase their sources of information on how to manage an affliction and in this way to enrich their knowledge about medicines, but they also do so to manage the risk associated with medicines and with the practice of self-medication, a point we will address below.

The information provided by the media also has an impact on the subjects' behaviour. But this impact can be unexpected. Thus, we can note the paradoxical effect produced for Nadine when she read a newspaper article that drew readers' attention to the dangerous nature of certain plants.[16] 'Even the most benign herbal teas should be handled with caution,' the article said. Nadine, who never used herbal medicine because she was not convinced of its efficacy, concluded, once warned about the potentially harmful effects of plants, that they must therefore necessarily also have a beneficial effect similarly to pharmaceuticals. She then decided, newly convinced of their power, to treat herself from then on with plants.

The knowledge individuals form of medicines and their use (indications, side effects, etc.) and the expertise that they gain from this, are thus forged at the intersection of these different sources of information. The question then remains as to the respective weight of these sources – which is the most valued and which will have the most influence on the concrete practices of ill people. On this point, it is striking to see how much, for all sources combined, some ill people attribute an importance to the recurrence of opinions, advice or accounts, basing their trust on the amount of agreement they find in these opinions. While the subjects' knowledge is composite – formed from knowledge transmitted by professionals, gained from their own experience and from accounts circulated on the Internet or transmitted by family, friends and acquaintances – an opinion becomes all the more valuable when it is confirmed by a second. Two identical accounts start to form a proof. Thus, the existence of at least *two* concurring opinions takes a decisive value, whether these are two opinions gathered on the Internet or one opinion on the Web coinciding with that of a family member or again an account of a person affected expressed on a forum corroborating with the personal experience of the web user reading it.

The knowledge the subjects acquire about drugs coexists with practices where the logic can differ radically from medical logic, but that the subjects nevertheless believe to be compatible with it. For example, when Josiane gets her medicines tested by a radiesthesist, the aim is to check whether the drug suits her well ('to see if they work for me', she explained), borrowing from the medical discourse that says a treatment should be adapted to an individual, to his/her organism and specific characteristics.

Ultimately, although an investigation into how individual knowledge is constituted in the context of self-medication appears to *a priori* amount to taking for granted that this knowledge is radically different from that of professionals, we can note that, in practising self-medication, the perception subjects have of these diverse forms of knowledge is far from being so entrenched and the boundaries are far from being so defined.

The issue of ill people's knowledge is regularly broached, not only to question their knowledge of therapies but also, beforehand, their ability to discriminate between benign and serious situations. In truth, knowing that individuals decide to self-medicate when their afflictions are benign does not tell us very much about what they consider to be benign nor does it address the problem of the boundary they set between benign situations and serious situations or pathologies.[17]

The assessment of the benign nature of an ailment, although based on experience, does not necessarily confer any knowledge. Indeed we can note that the experience is liable to promote a shift from 'lived situation' to 'known situation', and then to 'benign situation', according to a mechanism of convergence and assimilation. Liliane said she very rarely practices self-medication, except in cases she knows well. It is in these conditions that she gives her son Celestene 'as soon as he feels a bit breathless', as we have seen, thinking she knows this medicine well and that she 'now knows what he needs'. Equally, Christian, an estate agent, said he treats himself for 'non-serious' afflictions and that he 'knows how to recognise them' because he has 'already had them', which leads him to take the remnants of antibiotic treatments that were prescribed to him during previous episodes of ENT disorders. Christian said he limits his use of self-medication to cases of benign afflictions, but, in practice, he takes recourse to self-medication for symptoms he 'knows' by having already experienced them, added to the fact that he already possesses the medicines he believes to be appropriate for the case. For the users, the criteria is not so much the benign character of the ailment but their experience of it.

What should we understand by the subjects' decisions to use medicines they claim to know? The first difficulty lies in the meaning attributed to the notion of 'knowing' a medicine, which is often reduced to knowing its indications but not its composition nor its risks. In this way, Christiane, who does not think she practices self-medication at all and believes the only medicines she takes on her own initiative to be very mild and harmless, in fact regularly takes a hypnotic, in ignorance of the toxicity of the molecule in question. For her part, Josiane, who said she never self-medicates, regularly takes paracetamol to combat her headaches and plays down the consequences of this, saying: 'oh that, it's nothing, you see, it's got Sandoz written on it, it's not even Doliprane!'[18] This information came from her doctor, she said, who told her that Sandoz medicines were 'mild, with no side effects'.

Moreover, there are two phenomena present here and it is partly the synergy of the two that constructs the modalities of self-medicinal use: the translation of *known* symptoms into *benign* symptoms, which leads to medicinal use in situations that are not necessarily benign; and the semantic shift that takes places from object to be treated (the symptom) to treating object (the medicine), so that the medicines come to be considered as 'benign' in the image of the symptoms for which they are taken.

It follows from this, on one hand, that self-medication spreads from situations the subjects consider to be *benign* to situations they think are *known*; in other words, they associate benign pathologies and known pathologies, just like benign symptoms and known symptoms, or those thought to be such. On the other hand, the notion of 'benign situations' tends to apply, for the users, to both the illnesses treated and the medicines used. Consequently, people unworriedly use pharmaceuticals that are not harmless once they start to use them to manage a situation they believe they know. We can recall that it was because Richard had heard from his doctor that his abdominal pains and constipation were linked to stress and because he was then prescribed tranquilisers, that, from then on, when he had stomach pains or he noticed a slowing in his bowel movements, he turned to self-medication – and he took tranquilisers to combat his stress – thinking he now knew this pain and that there was no longer any need to consult a doctor when it reappeared.

Beyond the fact that the knowledge transmitted, acquired or reinterpreted is reappropriated by each subject according to his/her own modalities and forms the basis of the knowledge he/she possesses on medicines (Britten, 1994, 1996; Fainzang, 2000; Lupton, 2003; Dumit and Greenslit, 2006; Cardol et al., 2006; Nouguez, 2007) and self-medication, the notion of 'knowledge' is very ambiguous here, if only because the knowledge of a medicine, gained through the experience an individual has had of it, does not *ipso facto* confer to it a benign character. The unworried use of tranquilisers by a subject who claims to know this medicine because it was once prescribed by a doctor does not render the practice harmless, even when this knowledge is based on the said doctor's assertion that it is benign.[19] The result of this is that there exists a great uncertainty concerning what is 'known' by the subjects, and the nature of this 'knowledge'.

Hybrid knowledge

We have here, therefore, the constitution of hybrid, composite knowledge, where different forms of experience and information combine and feed one another. So what impact does this have on the practice of self-medication?

Advice, a vector of knowledge?

We know how much the notion of 'advice' is important in the recommendations from government ministries and professional institutions alike, and that pharmacists repeatedly remind us of their role in this regard (as we saw in Chapter 1). A pharmacist, having moved house and sold the pharmacy she owned in the Parisian suburbs to set up shop in the capital, complained about the change in her clientele and regrets that her 'advisory' role is now barely acknowledged. She said:

> In the other area there were people from Mali and North Africa, it was great! They were respectful! Here, we are just minions. These people come to buy what they need, they don't ask anything. But our job is to give advice! But they know everything, these *bobos*![20] They have no respect. It's disgraceful. They never come to thank me for my advice. Over there, they brought me presents. It's not for the presents, I'm just saying!

But advice is also, as we have seen, sought after and dispensed among people who know each other (within an acquaintance network) or among strangers (on discussion forums).

Between the words of pharmacists, of acquaintances and of web users, what role does 'advice' play in the construction of knowledge? The information campaigns concerning self-medication or medicinal use in general repeatedly remind us of the need to ask a pharmacist for 'advice'. But the notion of *advice* is rather nebulous and has barely been problematised in anthropology. Because what indeed is advice? What is the difference between the advice provided by a family member and the value it is assigned (which is extremely variable, considering the credibility the subject gives to the informant's opinion depending on his/her place in the kinship network and the relationship the subject has with him/her), and the advice given by a pharmacist?

We should emphasise the ambiguity of the notion of advice in the uses made of it. From a medical point of view, we cannot assimilate the 'advice' of a health professional with that of a parent, colleague or neighbour. An opinion, once it is given by a pharmacist, takes the status of a recommendation, almost equivalent, in that it is given by a health professional, to a prescription – although with no possibility of reimbursement. However, a pharmacist's advice can be positioned, in the subject's eyes, as a complement or even a competitor to the advice of a family member or an anonymous web user. Although, according to Bond and Bradley, pharmacists are the preferred health professional in the field of self-medication and considered veritable experts on the subject of medicines (Bond and Bradley, 1996),[21] we can see, on examination of the empirical situations described above, that pharmacists are sometimes, in terms of their diagnostic and pharmaceutical knowledge, the object of distrust which reduces their advice to the level of an opinion, on the same level as the advice dispensed by the subject's family and friends.

Vera's story demonstrates this. She believed she was badly 'advised' by her pharmacist. He had suggested she take an antacid for gastric reflux when in fact she had an intestinal bacteria and so she thought that this advice had led to a delay in diagnosis and decided to no longer consult him when in pain, since she did not credit him with a knowledge superior to that of her colleagues. It is very likely that, if it had turned out to be relevant, the pharmacist's advice would have been considered as professional expertise (even a medical prescription) – the only difference being that it would not have had the legal status of a prescription. But here, the pharmacist's 'advice' became an opinion amongst others. Not only is knowledge constituted from sources of variable status, but it is the adequacy of the advice and thus the unfolding of a therapeutic episode that will confirm this knowledge and the status of its source. Consequently, while 'advice' can take the value of an expert recommendation when it is provided by a pharmacist acting as a health professional with authority in the pharmaceutical domain, it can conversely be perceived simply as an 'opinion', competing with that of family members, and this is even more the case since it comes as a complement to the multiple opinions the subjects collect from those around them. Asking for advice is thus a highly ambivalent expression from an anthropological point of view.

However, the pharmacist's advice sometimes amounts to a suggestion of purchase. Béatrice, who was suffering from diarrhoea, went to a pharmacy and asked for Imodium (a drug she knew since she had already taken it). The pharmacist, who did not have Imodium in stock, gave her Lacteol. Béatrice told him she would rather have Imodium, but the pharmacist replied, 'It's the same thing'. Reassured, Béatrice bought the Lacteol. For her, it meant that this was a generic drug and only differed in the brand name, when in fact it is not the same molecule: one contains loperamide, while the other product is simply lactic acid.[22] Therefore, a pharmacist's advice does not necessarily involve transmitting knowledge about a medicine.

Composite knowledge

This reconstitution of knowledge, based on the multiplication and the recurrence of opinions, contributes to shaping the subjects' knowledge and to building their practice of self-medication. The passion of many for homeopathy (*Anthropologie et Santé*, 2011) to be taken as self-medication often results from this mechanism. It is not rare for doctors, for their part, to develop a discourse about a given medicine fed by the experience of their patients and shaped by their accounts. Indeed this is also the case for homeopathic products to which the doctors are sometimes *a priori* hostile or indifferent, and which then benefit from an evolving image: the doctors' discourses are partly built from contact with patients whose accounts sometimes lead them to modify their ideas of a medicine and its efficacy and in this way express a circular knowledge (i.e. one that circulates between doctors and patients) (Fainzang, 2006).

It is this same mechanism that can lead a subject to reject a medicine prescribed. It is after having read various articles on drug side effects that Joseph began to question an unpleasant sensation he was experiencing – a tingling of the skin every time he took a bath. He made the hypothesis that it was the result of taking a medicine prescribed to him to treat a mictional disorder linked to an enlarged prostrate because the tingling started at the beginning of this treatment, and so he decided to stop taking the drug. When he did so, the tingling seemed to disappear. He resolved to discuss it with his doctor, happy to be able to 'teach him something'. Although in this case it was non-compliance, resulting in what we could call 'de-medication' rather than self-medication, the subject thought he had acquired a form of knowledge of this medicine through his own experience and hoped to be able to share it with his doctor, thus contributing to the circulation of knowledge.

Thus the subjects possess knowledge that is constituted by that obtained from health professionals, from family and friends, from the media or as a result of their own experience. As we have seen, these categories have porous boundaries since these sources of information and modes of diffusion intertwine. While, prior to self-medicating, the multiple sources of information influence the choice of medicine, following self-medication, the knowledge gained is, in its turn, circulated to those around the subject, or communicated to other web users, making it liable to generate other self-medication practices. As we can see, experience and information combine to form the knowledge on which the practice of self-medication is based. The subjects' knowledge is a combination of knowledge from multiple sources since numerous forms of knowledge are put to use in self-medication, some from knowledge provided by health professionals, while others from the subjects' experience: experience-based knowledge is added to, or even mixed with, knowledge transmitted by information, from professional sources or not, giving rise to a *blended* knowledge.

However, beyond the examination of the way subjects constitute knowledge, the question of their competence is a difficult one, if only because ill people's decisions do not necessarily correspond with medical logic. While the subjects may not be 'right' in healthcare terms (in other words, if their therapeutic choices sometimes go against biomedical rationality), they can nevertheless have 'their reasons' in social terms, since their choices could answer to social or relational logics (Massé, 1997; Fainzang, 1997, 2001a). But additionally, the subjects can develop their therapeutic behaviours based on symbolic logics they borrow, or think they are borrowing, from medical logic. As we will discuss further in Chapter 5, the subjects' knowledge on which they base their practice of self-medication is anchored in an internalisation of the expert discourse, albeit distorted, and is the object of reconstructions and reinterpretations.

While people's power is an important stake in the context of health democracy, their knowledge is an even more decisive one since the latter is what gives the former its social legitimacy. As the object of conflicts and privileges, their knowledge is therefore, even more than the law, likely to serve and establish their power.

Notes

1 We will return to these notions later.
2 A mechanism indeed invoked in some traditional African societies to legitimise traditional practitioner knowledge (cf. Turner, 1967; Pouillon, 1977; Fainzang, 1986).
3 That is, the impression it makes on the sensory organs.
4 Guerci *et al.* (2002) showed that the exterior presentation is the first contact the user has with the medicine and that it transmits numerous messages, even if these are often unconciously assimilated.
5 Independently from any judgement of this practice that could be made from a medical point of view.
6 Excluding as such any type of medicine that is resistant to experimentation, such as homeopathy.
7 This is the case for Denise, who experimented with the consumption of chocolate to verify a potential sugar 'allergy'.
8 Trebaol *et al.* (2011) also underlined the limitations of this campaign but for other reasons.
9 That is, for not long enough.
10 Such as the knowledge passed on by the 'disseminator' in the *Vie libre* movement (Fainzang, 1996). See also Rabeharisoa and Callon (1999); Rabeharisoa (2008).
11 There she also learnt however that, as its origin was still not entirely certain, some sites advised people to pass their accounts onto to the anti-poison centre that is researching the cause of this phenomenon.
12 http://forum.doctissimo.fr/nutrition/allergies-alimentaires/gout-bouche-pignons-sujet_1225_1.htm
13 'If they say so on the telly, it is because it's true! It's not like information in a newspaper, it's not the same! A newspaper article is read by a thousand people at most whereas on the telly, there are millions of people who hear it! They can't just say whatever they like!'

14 It is striking to note in this regard the discrepancy, revealed by a Finnish study, between the sources of information used by parents practicing family medication for their children and the credibility they assign to these same sources (Hameen-Anttila *et al.*, 2010). The study showed that the sources of information the parents said they used the most were: doctors (72 per cent), drug information leaflets (67 per cent), nurses (52 per cent), and pharmacists (44 per cent); but that the parents considered the most reliable information sources to be doctors (50 per cent), drug information leaflets (31 per cent), nurses (37 per cent) and pharmacists (27 per cent). The discrepancy between these figures suggest that some sources of information are used without people believing them to be very reliable.

15 For this reason learning to critically read information on the Internet is vital not only for all patients within the framework of health education but for all individuals within the more general framework of citizen education.

16 'When medicinal herbs are poison. The Russian roulette of Chinese plants.' *Le Nouvel Observateur*, no. 1999, 27 February 2003.

17 It is precisely this difficulty in determining the benign nature of an affliction that the doctors evoke as a foundation for their hostile position towards self-medication, emphasising in particular the risk involved in a 'delay in diagnosis'.

18 Here there is confusion between the brand name and the pharmaceutical, since the paracetamol marketed by the Sandoz laboratory is the same molecule as that marketed by Sanofi under the brand name Doliprane.

19 We will return to this point for the case of Lexomyl (Chapter 5) that the subjects claim to know and which they state is harmless, and this is even more the case since the stick is breakable.

20 This word is a contraction of Bourgeois Bohemian. In France, it is a pejorative term for the leftist wealthy class.

21 However, we can assess the difficulty the users can have in building their trust in the health professionals from whom they should seek advice when the pharmacists advise them to take a certain treatment for a sore throat for example, but at the same time they read papers by pharmacologists based on hundreds of scientific publications saying that the non-prescription drugs sold for sore throats are totally ineffective. (See Giroud, 2011, whose work, aimed at the general public, was written in the style of a practical guide to non-prescription medicines.)

22 It should be noted that, according to Giroux (2011), the French National Health Authority considers Lacteol to be ineffective.

References

Aïach P. and Cèbe D., 1991, *Expression des symptômes et conduites de maladie*, Paris: Editions de l'Inserm/Doin.

Akrich A., Barthe Y. and Rémy C. (eds), 2010, *Sur la piste environnementale. Menaces sanitaires et mobilisations profanes*, Paris: Presses des Mines (coll. sciences sociales).

Akrich M., 1995, 'Petite anthropologie du médicament', *Techniques et culture*, 25-26: 129–157.

Akrich M. and Méadel C., 2002, 'Prendre ses médicaments / prendre la parole: les usages des médicaments par les patients dans les listes de discussion électroniques', *Sciences Sociales et Santé*, 20, 1 (special issue : 'Les médicaments: des prescriptions aux usages'): 89–116.

Akrich M. and Méadel C., 2004, 'Problématiser la question des usages', *Sciences Sociales et Santé* 22, 1 (special issue: 'Les technologies de l'information à l'épreuve des pratiques'): 5–20.

Anthropologie and Santé, 2011, 2, 'Anthropologie des soins non conventionnels du cancer' [http://anthropologiesante.revues.org/147].

Balcou-Debussche M., 2006, *L'éducation des malades chroniques. Une approche ethno-sociologique*, Paris: Editions des archives contemporaines.

Blech J., 2005, *Les inventeurs de maladies. Manœuvres et manipulations de l'industrie pharmaceutique*. Paris: Actes Sud (Babel).

Bond C.M., and Bradley C., 1996, 'Over the counter drugs: the interface between the community pharmacist and patients', *BMJ*, 312: 758–760.

Britten N., 1994, 'Patients' ideas about medicines. A qualitative study in a general practice population', *British Journal of General Practice*, 44: 465–468.

Britten N., 1996, 'Lay views of drugs and medicines: orthodox and unorthodox accounts', in: S.J. Williams, and M. Calnan (eds), *Modern medicine. Lay perspectives and experiences*, London: UCL Press.

Cardol M., Groenewegen P.P., Spreeuwenberg P., Van Dijk L., van den Bosch W.J. and De Bakker D.H., 2006, 'Why does it run in families? Explaining family similarity in help-seeking behaviour by shared circumstances, socialisation and selection', *Soc. Sci. Med.*, 63, 4: 920–932.

CSA/CECOP, 2007, 'Les Français et l'automédication', enquête exclusive réalisée pour la Mutualité Française.

Dumit J. and Greenslit N., 2006, 'Informated health and ethical identity management', *Culture, Medicine and Psychiatry*, 30, 2: 127–134 (special issue: 'Pharmaceutical Cultures').

Fainzang S., 1986, *'L'intérieur des choses'. Maladie, divination et reproduction sociale chez les Bisa du Burkina*. Paris: L'Harmattan.

Fainzang S., 1996, *Ethnologie des anciens alcooliques. La liberté ou la mort*. Paris: Presses Universitaires de France.

Fainzang S., 1997, 'Les stratégies paradoxales. Réflexions sur la question de l'incohérence des conduites de malades', *Sciences Sociales et Santé*, 15, 3: 5–23.

Fainzang S., 2000, *Of malady and misery. An Africanist perspective of illness in Europe*, Amsterdam: Het Spinhuis Publishers (Coll. Health, Culture and Society).

Fainzang S., 2001a, 'Cohérence, raison et paradoxe. L'anthropologie de la maladie aux prises avec la question de la rationalité', *Ethnologies comparées*, 3 [http://recherche.univ-montp3.fr/cerce/idx1.htm#F]

Fainzang S., 2006, 'Transmission et circulation des savoirs sur les médicaments dans la relation médecin-malade', in: J. Collin, M. Otero and L. Monnais (eds), *Le médicament au coeur de la socialité contemporaine. Regards croisés sur un objet complexe*, Montréal: Presses de l'université du Québec, 267–279.

Fox N.J., Ward K.J. and O'Rourke A.J., 2005, 'The "expert patient": empowerment or medical dominance? The case of weight loss, pharmaceutical drugs and the Internet', *Social Science and Medicine*, 60, 6: 1299–1309.

Friedson E., 1984, *La profession médicale*. Paris: Payot ('Médecine et sociétés').

Garro L., 2000, 'Cultural knowledge as resource in illness narratives: remembering through accounts of illness', in: C. Mattingly and L. Garro (eds). *Narrative and the cultural construction of illness and healing*, Berkeley: University of California Press.

Giddens A., 1991, *Modernity and self-identity*, Cambridge: Polity Press.

Giroud J.-P., 2011, *Médicaments sans ordonnance, les bons et les mauvais*, Paris: Ed. de la Martinière.

Good B.J., 1998, *Comment faire de l'anthropologie médicale? Médecine, rationalité et vécu*. Le Plessis-Robinson: Institut synthélabo pour le progrès de la connaissance.

Guerci A., Consigliere S. and Spinelli G., 2002, 'Médicament, emballage, écriture', communication au Colloque international de l'Amades: 'Anthropologie du médicament', Aix en Provence, 21–23 March 2002.

Hameen-Anttila K., Holappa M., Vainio K.and Ahonen R., 2010, 'What information sources do parents use when medicating their children?', from the 16th International Social Pharmacy Workshop, 'Communication and information in pharmacy', Lisbonne, 23–26 août 2010.

Hardey M., 2001, "'E-health'": the Internet and the transformation of patients into consumers and producers of health knowledge', *Information, Communication and Society*, 4, 3: 388–405.

Hardey M., 2004, 'Internet et société : reconfigurations du patient et de la médecine ?', *Sciences sociales et santé*, 22, 1: 5–20.

Hunter, N.D., 2010, 'Rights talk and patient subjectivity: the role of autonomy, equality and participation norms', *Georgetown Law Faculty Publications and Other Works*. Paper 473. [http://scholarship.law.georgetown.edu/facpub/473].

Jonville A.-P. and Autret E., 1994, 'Les erreurs d'utilisation des médicaments en pédiatrie: étude française prospective,' in: *L'enfant, sa famille et les médicaments*, Paris: Institut de l'Enfance et de la Famille, 95–97.

Jouet E., Flora L. and Las Vergnas O., 2010, 'Contruction et reconnaissance des savoirs expérientiels des patients: Note de synthèse', *Pratiques de formation/Analyses*, 57, 2010 (special issue: 'Usagers-Experts: la part du savoir des malades dans le système de santé'): 13–94.

Karsenty S., 1994, 'L'enfant, sa famille et les médicaments : approche sociologique et anthropologique', in: *L'enfant, sa famille et les médicaments*, Paris, Institut de l'Enfance et de la Famille, 41–49.

Karsenty S., 2009, 'Le retour hétéro-déterminé de l'automédication', *Sociologie Santé*, 30: 101–117.

Katz J., 1984, *The silent world of doctor and patient*, NY/London: The Free Press.

Laure P., 1998, 'Enquête sur les usagers de l'automédication: de la maladie à la performance', *Thérapie*, 53, 2: 127–135.

Lupton D., 2003, 'The lay perspectives on illness and disease', in: *Medicine as culture. Illness, disease and the body in western societies*. London/Thousand Oaks/New Delhi: Sage Publications.

Massé R., 1997, 'Les mirages de la rationalité des systèmes ethnomédicaux', *Anthropologie et Sociétés*, 21, 1: 53–71.

Mechanic D., 1980, 'The experience and reporting of common physical complaints', *Journal of Health and Social Behavior*, 21: 146–155.

Naraindas H., 2006, 'Of spineless babies and folic acid: evidence and efficacy in biomedicine and ayurvedic medicine', *Social Science and Medicine*, 62: 2658–2669.

Nouguez E., 2007, 'Copies conformes, comportements conformes? Les patients français face au choix des médicaments génériques', *Sociologie santé*, 26 ('Système de santé et discours profanes'): 247–261.

Pouillon J., 1977, *Fétiches sans fétichismes*. Paris: Maspero.

Rabeharisoa V. 2008, 'Experience, knowledge and empowerment: the increasing role of patients organizations in staging, weighting and circulating experience and knowledge. State of the art', in: M. Akrich, J. Nunes, F. Paterson and V. Rabeharisoa (eds), *The dynamics of patient organizations in Europe*, Paris: Presses des Mines, 13–34.

Rabeharisoa V. and Callon, M., 1999, *Le pouvoir des malades. L'Association française contre les myopathies et la Recherche*. Paris: Presses de l'Ecole des mines.

Renahy E., 2008, *Recherche d'information en matière de santé sur Internet: déterminants, pratiques et impact sur la santé et le recours aux soins*, Thèse de doctorat, Université Pierre et Marie Curie.

Renahy E., Parizot I., Lesieur S. and Chauvin P., 2007, *WHIST: Enquête web sur les habitudes de recherche d'informations liées à la santé sur Internet*, Paris: Inserm U707, 20 p.

Romeyer H., 2008, 'TIC et santé : entre information médicale et information de santé', *tic et société*, 2, 1 [http://ticetsociete.revues.org/365].

Thoër C., Pierret J. and Lévy J.J., 2008, 'Quelques réflexions sur des pratiques d'utilisation des médicaments hors cadre médical', *Drogues, santé et société*, 7, 1: 19–54.

Topçu S., Cuny C. and Serrano-Velarde K. (eds), 2008, *Savoirs en débat. Perspectives franco-allemandes*, Paris: L'Harmattan.

Tourette-Turgis C., 2010, 'Savoirs de patients, savoirs de soignants. La place du sujet supposé savoir en éducation thérapeutique', *Pratiques de formation/Analyses*, 57, 2010 (special issue: 'Usagers - Experts : la part du savoir des malades dans le système de santé'): 137–153.

Trebaol E., Haxaire C. and Bail P., 2011, 'Conceptions profanes de l'usage des antibiotiques et reception de la campagne de santé publique "les antibiotiques, c'est pas automatique"', *Sociologie Santé* (special issue: 'Les professionnels de santé: entre institutions et usagers'), 33: 127–148.

Turner V.W., 1967, *The forest of symbols, aspects of ndembu rituals*. New York: Cornell University Press.

Wyatt S., Henvood H.A. and Platzer H., 2004, 'L'extension des territoires du patient: Internet et santé au quotidien', *Sciences sociales et santé*, 1: 45–68.

5 Risk management and the quest for efficacy

Self-medication and its risks

Every year, thousands of people die from medicinal side effects and tens of thousands are admitted to hospital for the same reason.[1] The risk associated with medicinal use is clearly not the preserve of self-medication since it is also present for prescribed medicines (Lecomte, 1994; Rose, 2005, 2006; Dumit and Greenslit, 2006; Lakoff, 2006; Collin, 2007a, 2007b; Carricaburu, Castra and Cohen, 2010). Medicinal intake not only carries the risk of drug dependence as for psychoactive drugs – about which Giddens (1991) highlighted the dependencies induced in individuals using psycho-active substances within the framework of a medical prescription – but it also carries a risk of intoxication, as shown by a study of errors in medicinal use carried out at 15 anti-poison centres (Jonville and Autret, 1994). According to this study, out of 1108 errors recorded during a 6-month period, 31.5 per cent were the result of self-medication while 30 per cent were caused by an incorrect administration of a prescription and involved both users and professionals (pharmacists, doctors, nurses). These errors resulted from badly written, badly understood or badly administered prescriptions. Therefore, since the incorrect administration of a prescription implies the existence of a prescription in the first place, the failures and the dangers of medicinal intake go way beyond the framework of self-medication.

Non-informed drug use is of course likely to amplify the phenomenon. This is the reason that many doctors condemn self-medication, fearing the practice will increase these figures (Queneau, 1999). Indeed, the reason the health professionals, the public authorities and the pharmaceutical industry all agree in wanting to limit individual management to benign situations is precisely to mitigate this risk. They attempt to prevent not only the risk of an erroneous diagnosis or a delay in diagnosis (when personal management of the affliction leads the subjects to defer consulting a doctor) but also that of incorrect medicinal use.

The public debate surrounding self-medication, and especially open access, is thus largely structured around the issue of the risk contained in this practice and conceived to be inversely proportional to the user's competence. We would be wrong to think, however, that the subjects are not aware of these risks, or that they differ radically on this point from health professionals (Britten, 1994, 1996; Thoer-Fabre et al., 2007; Thoer, 2010; Fainzang, 2005, 2014; Hammer, 2010).

The users also harbour fears about self-medication. These fears are what prevent some people from practicing it, and what leads those who do so to try to reduce the associated risks. Here we will examine the modalities of risk management by the users of self-medication.

The availability of medicines   whether stored at home in a domestic medicine cabinet (Dew et al., 2014), or as over-the-counter products in a pharmacy – evidently makes self-medication easier simply by the proximity of the drugs and their physical accessibility. This availability, as a bearer of potential danger, forms the main argument of its detractors. The risk specific to self-medication is seen to reside in an incorrect understanding of the nature and the dosage of a medicine taken in response to a given pathological episode, and simply replicating a previous prescription does not succeed in eliminating this. Health professionals argue that any given case cannot be identical to the case for which a prescription has been given previously, despite what the subjects may presume. What can then ensue would be qualified by these professionals as *misuse*. While the brunt of the criticism in the literature is borne by cases concerning the misuse of psychoactive drugs (Fox et al., 2005; Thoer et al. 2008), it is also observable for many other types of medicine. Misuse, referring to an incorrect use carried out on the subjects' own initiative, often consists however of simply reproducing medical prescriptions. This often occurs with prescriptions of tranquilisers and antidepressants, profusely given by GPs,[2] on which subjects sometimes rely (as Mireille does; her doctor prescribed her the antidepressant, Deroxat, some years previously to overcome a period of depression following a break-up, which she now takes regularly to ensure she gets enough sleep).

Within the framework of self-medication, the use of psychoactive drugs is frequently problematic, whether it is inspired by a previous prescription or not, if only because these drugs are widely used as hypnotics even when this is neither their function nor their indication. Mr C, a chartered accountant, takes Lysanxia (a tranquiliser) on his own accord whenever he has to 'cope with stressful times at work' that affect his sleep. Although he was being treated by doctors for renal impairment and allergies, he said he did not want to 'delegate' his health to doctors for what he calls 'nervous tension problems'. Thus, the choice to self-medicate sometimes applies to specific pathological or bodily domains. Numerous psychoactive drugs are taken as hypnotics. This is the case for Lexomil, Temesta and Seresta, tranquilisers from the benzodiazepine family that are taken to resolve sleeping problems because of their sedative properties, and also for Noctran, which combines several active principles. Despite only being available with a medical prescription, they are frequently used in self-medication for this sole purpose. Evelyne regularly takes Temesta believing this drug to be a simple 'sedative'[3] that 'does no harm' since it is a 'tranquiliser'. The use of the terms 'tranquiliser' or 'anxiolytic' produce different social effects. In this regard, if we compare the information provided in the respective pharmaceutical leaflets, *Vidal* (for the doctors' use) and *Vidal for individuals* (for the patients' use), we can find that Lexomil is described as an 'anxiolytic' in *Vidal* and a 'tranquiliser' in *Vidal for individuals*. It is as if it is a matter of *tranquilising* patients who could be scared by the word *anxiolytic* and end up refusing to take the drug. Admittedly, the explicit aim of

Vidal for individuals is to 'promote better prescription compliance', as explained in the foreword. For some subjects however taking Lexomil is much less problematic than other similar drugs because they can break the stick into four parts (as the galenic preparation of this drug allows) thinking they have then eliminated any risk associated with repeated consumption.[4] This is the case for Mr R, a computer maintenance agent, who takes Lexomil on his own initiative to try to check what he calls his 'sweaty hand problem' – a bothersome sensation he experiences on various occasions. He has thus resorted to medicalising this bodily manifestation.

The argument of 'risk' (which borrows from the statistical register), or of 'danger' (which comes under the emotional register), is used in differing ways depending on the stance the actors take. The risk threshold, i.e. the moment at which the actors associate a self-medicinal practice with risk, is not always the same. But a dividing line does not only exist between the two categories of actors – the professionals and the users. It is also perceptible within the user category itself since their perception of risk is not homogenous; some tend to underestimate the risks (especially as regards open access drugs), while others develop strategies aiming to reduce them.

It is worth noting however that the argument of the risk contained in combining different active principles, invoked to condemn self-medication and presented by its opponents as the exemplification of incorrect medicinal use, is used in return by the subjects to question bad practice in the pharmaceutical industry when, upon noticing that the same molecule is marketed under different names, they realise that they have overdosed on one single substance when they thought they were taking two different ones. As such this issue engenders blame shifting, accusations and counter-accusations.[5]

Risk awareness

According to the definition proposed by Théophile and Bégaud (2009), pharmacovigilance 'brings together all activities aiming to detect, evaluate, quantify and prevent the adverse side-effects of commercialised medicines, and thus to optimise their risk-benefit ratio through appropriate decision-making, both individual and collective. These decisions encompass whether to prescribe a certain medicine or not, whether to adapt or stop a treatment, whether to modify the indication of the medicine or the information provided to doctors or patients, or even whether to withdraw the drug from the market' (p. 120). Upon consideration of this definition, we can see that, although pharmacovigilance is generally conceived as an activity carried out by professionals, the subjects too undertake, up to a certain point, a form of pharmacovigilance. They do so independently from ANSM's (the French Medicine and Health Product Safety Agency) encouragement to users to report any problems they have experienced with medicines,[6] by managing their medicinal consumption in a way that limits the associated risks. While it is not in their power to 'withdraw the medicine from the market', they can nevertheless decide to withdraw it from their shopping basket.

Indeed, people who practice self-medication are no more lacking in awareness of the risks involved than they are unaware of the risks associated with prescribed medicines. The 'scandals' concerning drugs with strong adverse side effects (where the controversy relates to them being put – and kept – on the market) have contributed to this awareness. They reinforce a suspicion not only towards the pharmaceutical industry suspected of concealing the risks inherent to a molecule, but also towards the medical discourse that is informed to a great extent by commercial campaigns and marketing communications from the pharmaceutical laboratories.

Risk awareness produces several types of reaction to self-medication, organised around two main models: either people refuse to practice it precisely because of the risks, or they decide to manage it in a way that limits them, because of the fear they induce. Fear is a powerful driver in decision-making and action in this domain: it organises the very practice of self-medication. Here it is not the illness that is feared, as for example when a subject fears his/her pathology may be serious which may lead him/her to prefer recourse to self-medication to avoid a consultation (Ostermann, 1999). This is a fear of the medicines themselves, which can be divided into different types: that of the secondary and adverse side effects of the substances, and that of drug interactions resulting from combining them, which together constitute the iatrogenic risks linked to medicinal intake. Fear of side effects, reinforced by reading pharmaceutical leaflets, limits or organises the practice of self-medication, just as it can hinder compliance to prescribed treatments.[7]

Fear thus plays a structuring role but has contrasting consequences. It structures both recourse and non-recourse to self-medication since it leads some people to abstain from the practice altogether. For these people, self-medication entails a reckless and potentially dangerous mix of chemical substances and they prefer to seek a medical consultation or even take recourse to alternative medicines. Pierre, a 40-year-old architect, never self-medicates. He does not think he is capable of doing so and prefers to consult a doctor if there is a 'problem' because he does not want to 'play the sorcerer's apprentice'. His attitude applies as much to choosing a treatment as to making a diagnosis or even undertaking a clinical examination: 'when the doctor asks me, "is it a dry cough or a chesty one?" I don't know! He's the one who should know.' Added to the fear of medicines and their effects, on which is based the desire to limit recourse to self-medication or even shun it altogether, is the fear of not being able to judge whether it is appropriate to take a certain medicine, linked to the fear of not being able to make the right diagnosis. So, the enthusiasm for autonomous health management is not shared by all.

Nevertheless, fear of medicines and fear of self-medication are not equivalent. Firstly, this is because the former can lead subjects to modify the dose, or even refuse to follow a prescription without actually renouncing self-medication in itself, and then, because the latter can sometimes lead subjects to refuse to self-medicate for ideological or political reasons, due to the taboo that continues to weigh on this practice in the eyes of a section of the population. One web user, who disapproved of self-medication, described it as 'the illegal practice of medicine'. The fear of self-medication and the refusal to take recourse to it are here induced by a social context, which defines the rights and powers of doctors *versus* those of patients. It then corresponds to a fear of performing a deviant act, sustained by the political dimension of self-medication.

On the other hand, subjects can wish to undertake an autonomous management of their health without however resorting to self-medication, for the very reason that they fear the medicines and their danger. Thus, Véronique uses non-medicinal techniques as much as possible to manage her affliction:

> I treat my pain by placing my hands on it; heat heals; I have learnt some Reiki.[8] It is less harmful than medicines! I discovered that when studying parapsychology in 1992. I can do regressions from birth and even before that. I managed to heal my friend's daughter who had terrible eczema; she had tried everything, but it wouldn't go away! And well, I did a regression on her, and she found an incestuous grandfather in her memories. And now, she is healed! No need to take medicines – cortisone and the like!

As we can see, subjects can manage an affliction and their health without this being self-medication.[9] While self-medication is a form of self-management, self-management on the other hand does not necessarily involve self-medication.

By contrast, fear nourishes in some people a desire to acquire enough knowledge about medicines to be able to manage their intake, or to have the tools available to verify their compatibility. And finally, it incites the subjects to develop strategies aiming to reduce these risks.

Patient strategies in the face of risk

The desire to know about the risks of a medicine leads subjects to take various precautions, such as gathering opinions or inquiring about the potential harmful effects of a drug from people they know (family, friends, colleagues, neighbours), whose unfortunate experience may incite caution. For example, Elodie is reluctant to take anti-inflammatories for her lumbar pain since her husband suffers violent stomach pains when he takes them, and so she prefers to use analgesics. The experience of animals can also be included. This is the case for Philippe, a 42-year-old industrial designer, who although little disposed to self-medication chose to take an antiemetic with confidence because he had once given it to his dog, and so he is now assured of the absence of harmful effects. In return, the subjects' personal experiences are passed on to those they dispense advice and recommendations to. The opinions gathered in the social network (family, friends and colleagues) thus complement or compete with opinions gathered on the Internet. We saw above the role played by the Internet in the constitution of knowledge, as one of several sources of information. But the knowledge acquired does not only relate to the existence of a certain medicine for a certain indication. Whether through medical sites or discussions undertaken on forums on the Web, Internet consultation provides details on the precautions to take and the conditions to respect to guarantee that the medicines do no harm. It is also in order to gather other people's experiences that a growing number of users browse the discussion forums, without necessarily participating themselves, in the hope of finding a description of a pathological situation similar to theirs and being able to identify with it. The aim is to benefit from other users' experience, although anonymous, on the effects of a medicine and whether they are satisfied or not or, inversely, on the potential set-backs of taking a certain drug. One user thus explained her problem and asked for an opinion on a forum with following question: 'Is it possible to take Doliprane at the same time as Zelitrex? I have herpes on my lip which is very painful and a split-ting migraine. I am desperate, please reply.'[10] Opinions expressed on forums can sometimes replace those of a pharmacists, either because the affliction is embar-rassing (a pharmacy does not lend itself to intimate talk about the body and users can experience difficulties in verbalising certain questions) or because it is more convenient (the advice arrives quicker), or simply to gain multiple points of view.

The perception of risk does not only depend on the perception a subject has of a medicine but also on *what* the medicine *is*. For example, some subjects claim to be against the consumption of psychoactive drugs but nevertheless, as we have seen, choose to take tranquilisers to solve sleeping problems (whether for difficul-ties in getting to sleep or night waking). The awareness of risk associated with medicinal intake through self-medication requires an acknowledgement of the fact that a medicine carries risk as soon as it has an action. Yet, some users do not consider a medicine to be risky if it is not a synthetic product. This goes for herbal medicines with which some subjects freely practice self-medication without cau-tion despite the potentially noxious effects of their use, just like other medicines. Or indeed, some medicines are not considered risky if their consumption is not intended to solve a health problem. This is the case for drugs taken 'to lose weight' that several patients believe are not 'real medicines' but simply cosmetics. Thus Mrs M (47 years old) claims to never practice self-medication ('I take things to lose weight, but they are not medicines') and does not distinguish between nutri-tional supplements based on green tea and weight-loss drugs. The definition of a medicine here depends on the purpose for which it is consumed.

Although the subjects do not always know about the specific risks of a drug, many of them know about the general, theoretical or potential risks, and adopt var-ious strategies aiming to minimise them. Beyond the social differences between individuals, which led Peretti-Watel (2001) to remark that their perception of risk is linked to the feeling of vulnerability, itself linked to their level of resources, self-medication almost always goes hand in hand with risk management, which borrows from varied cognitive systems. Even antibiotics – for which the high con-sumption in France is generally blamed on the patients' supposed enthusiasm for this type of drug – are the object of fear for subjects, without them knowing exactly what they should be afraid of. We can see this in the campaign about antibiotics discussed above, since, although they do not know what the risk of abusing anti-biotics actually is, some people nevertheless develop strategies aiming to mitigate it by reducing the number of days they take the medicine for, whether prescribed or taken as self-medication. It is precisely because of this concern to not overcon-sume antibiotics that they think it is reasonable to reduce the amount of time the medicine is taken for. This strategy is, for them, a response to the instruction to not abuse this type of drug, circulated by the health authorities. Therefore, they may lack knowledge of the type of risk they are taking by increasing the likelihood of antibiotic resistance, but they do not lack awareness of the risks associated with excessive consumption.

Risk *in itself* and risk *for oneself*

The strategies the subjects deploy differ according to whether they consider the risk to be inherent to the substance itself or linked to an uncontrolled use of the medicine. In the first case, the subjects tend to eliminate the product from the medicines they use (see Gérard's case or Elodie's attitude to anti-inflammatories). In the second, they attempt to neutralise the risks by modifying the recommended doses or the modes of consumption, whether in reference to a dosage recommended in the patient information leaflet or in a previous medical prescription.

The fear of drug interactions results in a decision to limit the number of medicines taken at a time. Fearing the consequences of taking chemicals that could produce harmful effects when combined and mixed, Nicole, 46 years old, believes that the number of medicines consumed should be limited, so she only consumes three substances at any one time. 'Once you take more than three, there are risks of illness, of interference,' she explained. Just as she chooses to take the medicines from her prescriptions that appear to her to be the most necessary without going over the number three, she also limits her self-medication in order to reduce the risk of medicinal interactions. Reducing the number of medicines to be taken at one time is based on a quantitative logic, the iatrogenic risk being linked to the quantity more than the quality of the types of pharmaceutical. This decision, which refers to a logic that is not validated by biomedical thought, is equivalent to a risk management strategy based on a personal assessment of the means of avoiding the risk.

A desire to limit medicinal risks also leads subjects to closely observe their effects in order to attempt to adapt the doses to their bodies, in recognition of a relationship between the medicine and the individual, in its singularity. 'I will need more than that! I am pretty tough,' said Julien, a company manager; whereas Noémie explained: 'I only take a tiny bit, less than they say in the leaflet, because I am very responsive to medicines.' These adaptations lead individuals to choose to increase or decrease the dosage (whether recommended in the pharmaceutical leaflet, advised by a pharmacist or prescribed during a previous consultation) when they deem the quantity to be inappropriate to their specific case. Alongside the reasoning that dictates the *quantity* of medicines to be taken figures another mechanism, which governs the choice of type or the *quality* of the medicines to consume. The risk then lies in the nature of the medicine, in the molecule contained in its composition and in the danger represented by its uncontrolled ingestion, in other words, in its qualitative aspect. This is what leads subjects to rule out, sometimes definitively, some classes of product (such as anti-inflammatories for example) from their choice of medication.

The strategies are therefore organised according to whether the risk is perceived as linked to the nature of the medicine in itself (the type of pharmaceutical product, their adverse side effects on certain functions or certain organs), or to its incompatibility with the subjects (in relation to their personal characteristics, or their drug absorption capacity, sensitivity, susceptibility or responsiveness, etc.). Philippe made sure his dog responded well to the antiemetic before he took it because of the risk *in itself* of a medicine. On the other hand, Josiane relies on a radiesthesist to make sure a medicine suits her and is appropriate to herself and her body because of the risk of the medicine *for oneself*. Risk management associated with the practice of self-medication thus follows multiple logics that are largely organised around the duality between the risk of the medicine *in itself* and the risk of the medicine *for oneself*.

Validation logics

Of course, the strategies the subjects develop to reduce the risk or maximise the efficacy of a treatment sometimes totally elude scientific logic. For example, the use of a radiesthesist's pendulum is a technique of validation from a decidedly non-scientific field. However, the intention here is not to differentiate between 'good' and 'bad' practices of risk management but to understand the symbolic logics to which this risk management relates and the mechanisms according to which it is elaborated. A notable aspect in this case is, first of all, the application of a non-scientific method to a biomedical product. The issue of therapeutic efficacy is generally perceived in anthropology in a context of 'medical pluralism' to mean recourse to plural institutions and health systems (for example Wallach, 2008). But the coexistence of several thought systems does not only lead to the use of therapies stemming from heterogeneous medical systems. In the context of self-medication, a subject can take recourse to a biomedical therapy (by using a biomedical medicine) but use a validation technique aiming to test its suitability or efficacy that borrows from a different system of thought. When Josiane has her medicines 'tested' by a radiesthesist to verify their safety and efficacy, she takes recourse to a technique from the domain of sensitivity that evades, as rhabdomancy does, biomedical rationality. Therefore, she is not assessing a medicine originating from alternative medicines but evaluating a synthetic product with alternative methods.[11] This act thus falls at the intersection of two systems: the biomedical system (with her use of a synthetic product) and a belief system linked to the domain of sensitivity (with her use of radiesthesia) used to test the suitability of the product from the first system.

In addition, aside from the judgement a health professional may make about the rationality, or lack of rationality, of this type of practice in relation to biomedical convictions, we have here an example of a strategy that is both anchored in syncretic cultural logic and borrows from medical logic while distorting it. Equally, Philippe's decision to take an antiemetic after noting the absence of harmful effects on his dog is an approach that, although inappropriate, makes this self-medicinal practice a *proven* technique in his eyes. This is done using a mechanism that prioritises experience-based medicine over evidence-based medicine.

The search for efficacy

The users also develop strategies to maximise the efficacy of medicines (Naraindas, 2006). Thus, just as the doses prescribed by a doctor may be increased in order to strengthen their effects (Van der Geest and Whyte, 1988; Etkin, 1992), some medicines chosen for self-medication are taken at a higher dose than the recommended average specified in the pharmaceutical leaflet or indicated in a previous prescription.

In the same way as the absence of risk can be tested, the efficacy of a medicine is often, if not tested, at least deduced from experience. Here again, the experience that informs the decision to choose a certain drug can be that of the subject on a previous occasion, or that of a family member (even an animal), or that of an anonymous other (recounted on the Internet). It was because he saw his parents treating their dogs and chickens with homeopathy when he was a child that Paul now treats himself with homeopathy, the efficacy of which appears to him to have thus been demonstrated.

The complexity of the search for efficacy through medicinal use – a search that is sometimes similar to a true quest – lies in the fact that the drug indications do not necessarily match with their actual use. The use of medicines for non-therapeutic ends has been widely documented. Thoër *et al.*, 2008; Aubé and Thoër, 2010, for example, showed that some people use psychoactive drugs for recreational ends. However, inversely, substances that are not medicines can be used as such, through the means by which they are used. Subjects can consume certain foods for example in a very 'structured' way, following precise procedures in the manner of medicinal intake in order to extract maximum benefit. This occurs not only with dietary supplements (which, despite the fact that some professionals claim they are inefficacious,[12] are packaged, sold and consumed *in the same way as* medicines) but also with simple foodstuffs to which the subjects end up conferring a status close to that of a medicine through the use they make of them, within a framework of a quasi-ritual that is thought to increase their efficacy. Louise thus conscientiously eats an apple morning, noon and night, ever since she read an article on the numerous virtues of this fruit (antioxidant, digestive, etc.), while Thérèse, having learnt that one should drink enough water to prevent all sorts of pathologies (urinary infections, gallstones, dehydration), forces herself to drink a glass of water every two hours and never departs from this self-prescription. Scrupulous consumption of a substance (food, drink, etc.), every day at the same time, in a sort of routine based on a precise dosage (time of day, quantity taken), seems to guarantee in the subjects' eyes the maintenance of their health or the resolution of a deficiency.

What is the medical service rendered?

The practice of removing eligibility for reimbursement from medicines has engendered some dubious reactions from the users. Many users consider, to the despair of the pharmaceutical industry, that if the public authorities have removed this eligibility it is because the drugs in question are not efficacious. They object to buying such drugs when advised by their pharmacist, preferring a reimbursable medicine – even if they have to shoulder the cost themselves. To combat this interpretation of the removal of eligibility for reimbursement, the public authorities repeatedly specify that the drug's efficacy is not under question, but that said medicine has been removed from the list of reimbursable drugs because the medical service they render has been judged insufficient (HAS [French National Authority for Health], 2008). This medicinal policy is thus based on the notion of 'medical service rendered' (SMR: *service médical rendu*). Eligibility for reimbursement is removed from medicines once it is established that they do not render a sufficient medical service to justify public funding (HAS, 2008).[13] The question is then what this 'medical service rendered' covers exactly. For the public authorities, the SMR takes several aspects into account: the seriousness of the pathology for which the medicine is indicated, the data specific to the medicine (efficacy and side effects), the existence of therapeutic alternatives and its significance for public health. 'In accordance with the assessment of these criteria, several levels of SMR have been defined: major or important SMR, moderate or weak SMR that nevertheless justifies reimbursement, and insufficient SMR (SMRI) to justify public funding' (HAS, 2008).

The multiple aspects of the definition of the SMRI contribute to the ambiguity of this notion. In this regard, Claude Le Pen (2003) thought that 'the confusion between medicines that have had their eligibility for reimbursement removed and inefficacious medicines, harms medicines said to be for 'self-medication'.[14] He asked: 'If the SMR is judged insufficient for a certain medicine, why then is it only removed from the list of eligible drugs? It would be more in the public interest to purely and simply remove it from the market' (p. 48). Equally, the Journal *Revue Prescrire* (2008) believes that 'to guarantee self-medication that benefits patients, the first measure to be taken is the removal of any medicine from the market where the risk-benefit ratio is not favourable'. The question of why insufficiently effective drugs remain on the market remains highly pertinent today.[15]

What is at stake in this debate is the cognitive treatment of the notion of SMR. Is a medicine with a weak or insufficient SMR one that treats a pathology that is 'weakly' serious, or a medicine that treats a pathology with a 'weak' success rate? The industry understands the term in the first sense when it proposes a shift in the distinction between SMR and SMRI to encompass the distinction between serious and benign pathologies. The National Authority for Health however understands the concept in the second way. The public authorities specify that they are assessing the 'performance level' to determine whether a medicine should be reimbursed or not, and that the removal of eligibility for reimbursement is proposed for medicines 'whose funding is not the priority', and that a medicine is judged to have an insufficient SMR when 'the performance level of the drug is judged too weak to justify public funding' (HAS, 2008). We should note that the focus of the debate shifts depending on the terms used, since the cognitive cursor oscillates between types of medicines – with high/low performance, with high/low priority – and types of pathology – serious/benign. Consequently, if for the public authorities a medicine with an 'insufficient' SMR is not an 'inefficacious' medicine, it nevertheless has an 'insufficient performance'. But the users are not fooled: why then should they look to acquire the medicines with the lowest performance?

Between efficacy and safety

Modifying a prescribed treatment (increasing or decreasing doses, prolonging or shortening the treatment duration, etc.), which the health professionals deem to be poor compliance, could be considered to some extent as a form of self-medication consisting of reappropriating some medical knowledge but using this knowledge 'in an autonomous way' (Haxaire, 2001, in reference to psychoactive drugs). In describing a case of a patient who attributed his anxiety to certain events in his life and who decided to abruptly stop the tranquiliser treatment when his life circumstances changed without consulting his doctor, Haxaire thus widened the practice of self-medication to include the 'adjustment' of prescribed treatments.

Admittedly, common features exist between (what the doctors judge as) poor compliance and self-medication since, as we have seen, taking a prescribed treatment following a medical consultation can involve reassessing and reinterpreting the prescription, based on what the subjects believe to be relevant. Indeed, the subjects' reluctance to take some medicines as self-medication partly echoes the reluctance that leads them to poorly adhere to prescriptions. My previous research demonstrated that the anxiety induced by medicines differs depending on the categories of pharmaceuticals, the subjects and the cultural groups to which they belong (Fainzang, 2001b). This reluctance, which brings into play representations of the person and relates to diverse registers (physical, psychic, behavioural and social), is expressed in particular towards medicines suspected of having harmful effects on an organ, or of endangering the proper functioning of the body. Modifying a previously prescribed treatment (increasing or reducing the dose, prolonging or shortening the treatment duration, even refusing to take the medicine in question altogether) is most often the result of a previous negative experience of this treatment and its effects. This reluctance is likely to also curb any leaning the subjects may have towards choosing to self-medicate. Just as Gérard one day refused to follow a prescription of Nexen (an anti-inflammatory) that he tolerated badly, he also refuses to take anti-inflammatories as self-medication. In this regard, the attitude toward generics does not appear to differ between prescribed medicines and those taken as self-medication. The relationship the subjects maintain with generic medicines, whether this is one of distrust (Nouguez, 2007; Sarradon-Eck *et al.*, 2007) or trust, is the same *within* or *outside* a prescription. However, because the practice of self-medication induces subjects to read the pharmaceutical leaflets more thoroughly (although this is not systematic), the presence of a term such as 'excipient' often intrigues them. For them the word means 'there is something else' or 'something different', likely to induce an efficacy or a risk that is also different, echoing on this point the discourse of many doctors.[16]

In reference to how patients comply with their prescriptions, I highlighted the existence of various logics that underpin prescription modifications: a *cumulative logic*, consisting of increasing dosages or even accumulating several medicines in order to increase the chances of recovery, and an *identity logic*, consisting of modifying a treatment based on identifying a link between oneself and the product, whether one is (or considers oneself to be) fat or thin, strong or weak, adult or child, man or woman, resistant or frail, etc. (Fainzang, 2001b). I have shown that such logics partly inform the choice as to whether to adhere to or modify the doses prescribed.

These logics, which form the basis of the patients' reinterpretation of a medical prescription, also bear on how the medicines consumed within the framework of self-medication are managed. Thus we find cumulative logic and identity logic within the practice of self-medication, both in the search for better efficacy and in order to reduce the negative effects of medicines. Recommended doses, either from a previous consultation resulting in a prescription, from the patient information leaflet of a medicine or advised by a pharmacist, can thus sometimes be increased in order to boost efficacy, or in contrast, reduced to avoid inducing iatrogenic effects.

However, while self-medication has some affinity with the adjustment or modification of prescriptions or even with 'poor compliance', it involves even more marked changes since it necessarily involves a self-diagnosis, particularly when a doctor has not been consulted in the past for the same symptom. In this case, the subjects undertake the management of risk and the search for efficacy alone.

The definitions or redefinitions of treatments in self-medication are based on a logic the subjects perceive to be medical, in that they are convinced they are conforming to the precautions of use, and adapting their self-prescription to their body and their singularity (their age, sex, weight ...). The adaptation of previous prescriptions and/or the reduction of the dose indicated on the drug leaflet thus partly responds to the concern not to follow prescriptions where the doses are considered to be excessive, based on realigning the cumulative logic and the identity logic. Here we have mechanisms that, while they do not echo professional logics, do however stem from strategies destined to obtain an optimal medicinal use, borrowing from biomedical logic and seeking a balance between safety and efficacy.

Effects and efficacy

The existence of secondary or adverse side effects is not necessarily in itself an obstacle to self-medication (no more than it is necessarily an obstacle to prescription compliance). While it is true that reading about the side effects in pharmaceutical leaflets sometimes dissuades patients from taking the medicines prescribed,[17] the opposite can also apply where the subjects interpret their presence as a sign of genuine efficacy to the point that however 'adverse' this effect is, the subjects still do not envisage ending the treatment. The effects, good or bad, are a sign of its efficacy and prove the treatment should be continued, without the subjects seeing the possibility of any unfortunate consequences. For Mr B, 'a good medicine is one that does something'. Risk awareness is thus not always the same as knowing about the possible iatrogenic effects of the medicine.

On this point, the significance here lies in the nature of the effect in question more than in its 'secondary' or even 'adverse' character. The distinction between these two effects is far from clear for the users, considering the ambiguity of the notions in the pharmaceutical leaflets. While, strictly speaking, a secondary effect is a non-desired reaction, provoked by the administration of a medicine, in addition to the primary desired effect during the application of a treatment for a given indication, an 'adverse side effect' is a 'harmful non-desired reaction to a medicine, produced by normally used doses in man for the prophylaxis, diagnosis or treatment of a disease or for the recovery, rectification or modification of a physiological function'.[18] In this regard, listing the 'secondary effects' in a pharmaceutical leaflet makes the drug sound less negative than 'adverse side effects'. Indeed it is with this acceptation that the WHO intends them to be used. Yet, some medicines are chosen precisely for their secondary effects and not for the indication intended (as suggested by Etkin, 1992, or by Nichter and Vuckovic, 1994), making the secondary effect a desired effect as the primary one is. In this case, the secondary effect is no longer simply a sign of the drug's efficacy but the vector of a new efficacy, which leads to a medicinal use that is not linked to its indication but to its secondary effects or, we could say, for the very reason of the presence of these secondary effects. The secondary effect is then identified as a 'secondary benefit'.

The same phenomenon can be observed for *adverse side effects.* Some antihistamines (antiallergenics such as Polaramine, or cough medicines such as Toplexil) are sometimes taken as hypnotics precisely because of the drowsiness they can induce. Thus, Liliane uses Neo-codion to address her child's difficulties in getting to sleep; she believes the child is often overly excited in the evening. Although drowsiness is a 'possible adverse side effect' of the medicine, induced by the presence of codeine, it is used for this very reason and not for its indication as a cough medicine. Here the subjects choose the medicine because of its sedative qualities, their decision sometimes supported by the recommendation in the patient information leaflet to take the substance in the evening. This is also the case for Lexomil which, as we have seen, users often take not for the indicated use (which is a symptomatic treatment of manifestations of severe and/or incapacitating anxiety) but in order to induce drowsiness, considered to be one of the adverse side-effects of this medicine.[19] An *undesirable effect* can then become, as these uses demonstrate, a *desired effect.*[20]

As shown in this decoding of social practices, subjects deploy all sorts of strategies aiming to both minimise the risks associated with medicines and to maximise their effect. However, the subjects' perception of the risks and efficacy of medicines is sometimes very personal, and the assessment criteria belong to them alone. Their convictions are largely rooted in their past experience and rely on pragmatic mechanisms that transform the secondary effects of medicines into primary effects, and the undesirable side effects into desired effects.

In the strategies employed within the practice of self-medication there is thus a tension between two objectives: the search for efficacy and the prevention (or management) of risk. Safety and efficacy are considered simultaneously. Subjects tend to seek a balance between the two, that is to say, they seek an efficacy with minimal risk by applying a balancing principle. While the logics that underpin self-medication (the management of risk and the search for efficacy) partly resemble, as we have seen, those that underpin compliance (or non-compliance) with prescriptions, this balancing leans towards a different combination in that it integrates in an even more marked way the need for the subject to establish an appropriate relationship, in accordance with personal rationalities, between a given substance and his/her body. The practices linked to reducing risks and seeking efficacy are, to an even greater extent in self-medication, infused with symbolic logics.

The decision to modify the dosage of a treatment or to check the drug's compatibility with personal bodily characteristics, by means of what we have called *cumulative logic* and *identity logic*, or by means of the validation techniques mentioned above, is based on the interiorisation of learnt behavioural norms that are transmitted throughout the process of socialising patients by health professionals. The subjects are placed in a situation of being agents of an autonomous practice and are no longer patients, and so they adapt and *personalise* their treatment in order to increase its efficacy and reduce its risk.[21] The majority of health professionals themselves highlight the need for treatments to be adapted to an individual. One of the reasons they give for why people should ask for advice from pharmacists is precisely this fact: that each person reacts differently to medicines.[22] Although the methods of validation used by subjects are not endorsed by biomedicine, they respond to the norms and instructions diffused by medical thinking, namely that treatments should be personalised. As we can see, while their choices may be structured according to personal or collective symbolic and cultural logics, they also borrow from medical thinking, using strategies of validation, verification, experimentation and personalisation.

Notes

1 These figures are provided by the EMIR study (Adverse Side Effects of Medicines: Implications and Risks) that supplies up-to-date data on hospitalisations due to adverse side effects of medicines, the results of which are regularly diffused by the French Medicine and Health Products Safety Agency (ANSM).

2 80 per cent of psychoactive drugs taken in France are prescribed by GPs (Le Moigne, 1999), a practice condemned by many psychiatrists who believe such prescriptions are inappropriate.

3 On the perception of 'calming' drugs, see Haxaire (2001).

4 We can question however why the laboratory considers it preferable to present the drug in this way and not in pill form with a quarter of the current dosage, since health professionals often advise breaking the stick into four. The result is that many subjects tend to think that there is no harm in regularly taking a whole stick since ultimately that only amounts to taking one at a time.

5 The risk lies in describing medicines by their commercial name rather than their INN (International Non-proprietary Name), which is the substance name. For many users, the plurality of medicine names denotes a plurality of pharmaceutical specialities. This is the reason that the journal *Revue Prescrire* (2012) has been recommending the use of the INN for a long time, since the diversity of brand names gives rise to confusion.

6 'Report an adverse side-effect': http://ansm.sante.fr/Declarer-un-effet-indesirable/Comment-declarer-un-effet-indesirable/Declarer-un-effet-indesirable-mode-d-emploi/(offset)/0

7 Non-observance and self-medication share a certain amount of common ground, to which we will return further on. However, within the framework of self-medication, it

is not simply, or not necessarily, a case of making a judgement on the appropriateness of a previously prescribed treatment. It is in fact a case of judging *oneself* the suitability of a treatment.

8 A non-conventional medicine originating in Japan, based on energy healing by the laying-on of hands.

9 Equally, 'self-regulation', which for Pierret (2009) consists of appropriating a treatment, cannot be identified with self-medication since it corresponds to the second step in the process of integrating a prescribed treatment, after its 'acceptance'.

10 http://forum.doctissimo.fr/medicaments/medicaments-libre/

11 On unusual combinations of different medical systems, see *Anthropologie and Santé* (2011).

12 Giroud, 2011.

13 www.has-sante.fr

14 The problem of equating removal of eligibility for reimbursement with inefficacy was raised in the Coulomb Report itself. It proposed that 'the badly understood and harmful notion of a medicine with an 'insufficient SMR' should be abandoned and replaced with the term 'non-priority' medicines'. This latter notion however is no less ambiguous.

15 A question that Giroud (2011) also raised when he noted that the French National Authority for Health only assesses the medical service rendered for reimbursed products and that the marketing of medicines devoid of any proven efficacy is authorised (p. 26).

16 http://mon-medecin-m-a-dit.over-blog.com/article-27276959.html

17 This is what leads some doctors to hide or even deny the existence of such effects (Fainzang, 2015).

18 According to the official definition used by the WHO and the European Community.

19 A risk that appears in the leaflet alongside its opposite – that of insomnia.

20 We can note that the confusion between secondary and adverse side effects is compounded by the patient information leaflets where neuro-vegetative effects such as drowsiness, induced by some molecules, are sometimes mentioned among the secondary effects and sometimes among the adverse side effects.

21 In her investigation of the conditions of compliance in the context of hypertension, Sarradon-Eck (2007) showed that many subjects use the notion of compatibility between the medicine and the individual to explain the success or failure of a treatment, and that it is an important factor in their reluctance to take generic drugs, which according to them would obstruct this personalisation of the treatment.

22 A recommendation that goes way beyond our borders since it can also be found on a Canadian website: www.monpharmacien.ca/fr/questions-reponses/raisons-consulter.php

References

Anthropologie and Santé, 2011, 2, 'Anthropologie des soins non conventionnels du cancer' [http://anthropologiesante.revues.org/147].

Aubé S. and Thoër C., 2010, 'La construction des savoirs relatifs aux médicaments sur Internet: étude exploratoire d'un forum sur les produits amaigrissants utilisés sans supervision médicale', in: Lise Renaud (ed.) *Les médias et la santé: de l'émergence à l'appropriation des normes sociales*, Coll. « Santé et société », Québec: Presses de l'Université du Québec, 239–266.

Britten N., 1994, 'Patients' ideas about medicines. A qualitative study in a general practice population', *British Journal of General Practice*, 44; 465–468.

Britten N., 1996, 'Lay views of drugs and medicines: orthodox and unorthodox accounts', in: S.J. Williams, and M. Calnan (eds), *Modern medicine. Lay perspectives and experiences*, London: UCL Press.

Carricaburu D., Castra M. and Cohen P. (eds), 2010, *Risque et pratiques médicales*, Rennes: Presses de l'EHESP.

Collin J., 2007a, 'Relations de sens et relations de fonction: risque et médicament', *Sociologie et sociétés*, 39, 1: 99–122.

Collin J., 2007b, 'Du silence des organes au souci de soi: médicament et reconfiguration de la notion de prévention', in: I. Rossi (ed.), *Prévoir et prévoir la maladie. De la divination au pronostic*, Monts: Aux lieux d'être, 139–151.

Dew K., Chamberlain K., Hodgetts D., Norris P., Radley A. and Gabe J., 2014, Home as a hybrid centre of medication practice, *Sociology of Health & Illness*, 36, 1: 28–43.

Dumit J. and Greenslit N., 2006, 'Informated health and ethical identity management', *Culture, Medicine and Psychiatry*, 30, 2: 127–134 (special issue: 'Pharmaceutical Cultures').

Etkin N.L., 1992, '"Side effects": cultural constructions and reinterpretations of western pharmaceuticals', *Medical Anthropology Quarterly*, 6, 2: 99–113.

Fainzang S., 2001b, *Médicaments et société. Le patient, le médecin et l'ordonnance*, Paris: Presses Universitaires de France.

Fainzang S., 2005, 'Religious attitudes toward prescriptions, medicines and doctors in France', *Culture, Medicine and Psychiatry*, 29, 4: 457–476.

Fainzang S., 2014, 'Managing medicinal risks in self-medication', *Drug Safety*, 37, 5: 333–342.

Fainzang S., 2015, *An anthropology of lying: information in the doctor-patient relationship*, Farnham: Ashgate.

Fox N.J., Ward K.J. and O'Rourke A.J., 2005, 'The "expert patient": empowerment or medical dominance? The case of weight loss, pharmaceutical drugs and the Internet', *Social Science and Medicine*, 60, 6: 1299–1309.

Giddens A., 1991, *Modernity and self-identity*, Cambridge: Polity Press.

Giroud J.-P., 2011, *Médicaments sans ordonnance, les bons et les mauvais*, Paris: Ed. de la Martinière.

Hammer R., 2010, *Expériences ordinaires de la médecine. Confiances, croyances et critiques profanes*, Zurich/Genève: Ed. Seismo.

Haute Autorité de Santé [HAS], 2008, 'Prise en charge des médicaments soumis à réévaluation', [www.has-sante.fr].

Haxaire C., 2001, '"Calmer les nerfs": automédication, observance et dépendance à l'égard des médicaments psychotropes', *Sciences sociales et santé* (special issue: 'Les médicaments: des prescriptions aux usages'), 20, 1: 63–86.

Jonville A.-P. and Autret E., 1994, 'Les erreurs d'utilisation des médicaments en pédiatrie: étude française prospective,' in: *L'enfant, sa famille et les médicaments*, Paris: Institut de l'Enfance et de la Famille, 95–97.

Lakoff A., 2006, *Pharmaceutical reason. Knowledge and value in global psychiatry*, Cambridge: Cambridge University Press (Series: Cambridge Studies in Society and the Life Sciences).

Le Moigne Ph., 1999, *Anxiolytiques, hypnotiques. Les facteurs sociaux de la consommation*. Document of the GDR 'Psychotropes, Politique et Société', 1.

Le Pen C., 2003, *Automédication et Santé Publique: le 'Service médical rendu' par les médicaments d'automédication*, CLP-Santé Paris, report made in collaboration with l'AFIPA.

Lecomte T., 1994, 'La consommation pharmaceutique des enfants de moins de 10 ans d'après les données de l'enquête sur la santé et les soins médicaux réalisée en 1991–92', in: *L'enfant, sa famille et les médicaments*, Paris: Institut de l'Enfance et de la Famille, 55–68.

Naraindas H., 2006, 'Of spineless babies and folic acid: evidence and efficacy in biomedicine and ayurvedic medicine', *Social Science and Medicine*, 62: 2658–2669.

Nichter M. and Vuckovic N., 1994, 'Agenda for an anthropology of pharmaceutical practice', *Social Science and Medicine*, 39, 11: 1509–1525.

Nouguez E., 2007, 'Copies conformes, comportements conformes? Les patients français face au choix des médicaments génériques', *Sociologie santé*, 26 ('Système de santé et discours profanes'): 247–261.

Ostermann G., 1999, 'Aspects psychologiques de l'automédication', in: P. Queneau (ed.), *Automédication, autoprescription, autoconsommation*. Paris: John Libbey, 33–38.

Peretti-Watel P., 2001, *La société du risque*. Paris: La Découverte, coll. Repères.

Pierret P., 2009, 'De l'observance à l'intégration du traitement: pour une approche dynamique', in: C. Garnier C. and J.J. Lévy(eds), *Médicaments, de la conception à la prescription*, Montréal, Liber, 195–205.

Queneau P., 1999, 'Automédication en antalgiques', in: P. Queneau(ed.), *Automédication, autoprescription, autoconsommation*, Paris: John Libbey, 84–95.

Revue Prescrire, 2008, 'Médicaments en libre accès bientôt autorisés, sûrement pas obligatoires', 28, 295: 337.

Revue Prescrire, 2012, 'Ordonnance: la dénomination commune internationale (DCI) au quotidien', 32, 346: 586–591.

Rose N., 2005, 'In search of certainty: risk management in a biological age', *Journal of Public Mental Health*, 4, 3: 14–22.

Rose N., 2006, 'Disorders without borders? The expanding scope of psychiatric practice', *Biosocieties*, 1, 4: 465–484.

Sarradon-Eck A., 2007, 'Le sens de l'observance. Ethnographie des pratiques médicamenteuses de personnes hypertendues', *Sciences sociales et santé*, 25, 2: 5–36.

Sarradon-Eck A., Blanc M.A. and Faure M., 2007, 'Des usagers sceptiques face aux médicaments génériques: une approche anthropologique', *Revue d'épidémiologie et de santé publique*, 55: 179–185.

Théophile H. and Bégaud B., 2009, 'La pharmaco-épidémiologie ou l'évaluation du médicament dans la vie réelle', in: C. Garnier and J.J. Lévy (eds), *Médicaments, de la conception à la prescription*, Montréal: Liber, 105–124.

Thoër-Fabre C., Garnier C., Dufort F., Levy J.J., Beaulac Baillargeon L., 2007, 'Perceptions profanes des risques associés à l'hormonothérapie: un "bricolage" des savoirs', *Sociologie-Santé, 26*, 2: 227–245.

Thoër C., 2010, 'Risque médicamenteux et renégociation de la confiance au sein de la relation médecin-patient: Perspectives de médecins français et québécois sur la publication de la Women's Health initiative', *Sciences de la Société*, 76: 147–166.

Thoër C., Pierret J. and Lévy J.J., 2008, 'Quelques réflexions sur des pratiques d'utilisation des médicaments hors cadre médical', *Drogues, santé et société*, 7, 1: 19–54.

Van der Geest S. and Whyte S.R., 1988, *The context of medicines in developing countries*, Dordrecht: Kluwer Academic Publishers.

Wallach I., 2008, 'Automédication et pluralisme thérapeutique chez les jeunes d'origine chinoise vivant en France et au Québec', *Revue internationale sur le médicament*, 2: 139–185.

Conclusion

I began this book by underlining the changes in the current context regarding self-medication. While this practice was strongly discouraged in the past (Fainzang, 2001), it is today openly encouraged by the public authorities and some health professionals, and demanded by the users. The image of self-medication has been modified by both the transformations within the health system (Blenkisopp and Bradley, 1996) and the evolution of the status of ill people who are now considered to be autonomous subjects (see for instance Giddens 1987, 1991; Hoerni, 1991; Gagnon 1995, 1998; Rameix, 1997; Prayle and Brazier, 1998; Ikonomidis and Singer, 1999; Schneider, 1999; Mackenzie and Stoljar, 2000; Schneewind, 2001; Tristram Engelhardt, 2001; Rothman, 2001; Orfali, 2003; Meyers, 2004; CCNE, 2005; Pierron, 2007; Jouan and Laugier, 2009; Ehrenberg, 2009; Hunter, 2010; Baszanger, 2010). The practice of self-medication is now acceptable and permitted (at least in some situations), and subjects are invited to discuss it with their doctors without fear or reproach. The ten commandments of self-medication[1] recommend, on Vidal's website, *Eureka santé*,[2] that people should not practice 'shameful self-medication', which would involve hiding 'unsuccessful attempts at self-medication' from the doctor; they are instead encouraged to reveal the treatments taken 'under one's own initiative' to relieve 'minor ailments'.

To some extent, Aïach and Cèbe's observation in 1991 was correct. They wrote that 'the nature of the medical system in place greatly influences whether self-medication comes to substitute medical consumption or not' (p. 11). After Lecomte (1988, 1999), they also rightly used 'the existence of a public health system that allows the majority of individuals to be reimbursed for most of their medical costs and that encourages people to consult a doctor to obtain a prescription and medicinal reimbursement' to explain the fact that self-medication did not appear to be used as an alternative to medical consultation. Indeed, inversely, the changes in the medicinal reimbursement system in France today are likely to stimulate self-medication.

However, the development of this practice cannot be solely explained by economic considerations. The context of health democracy, claims of 'patient power' and the development of individual autonomy linked to the expansion of the Internet and the increase in individual sources of information have contributed to making the practice more commonplace and democratic. In the face of this, the subjects, commonly called 'expert-patients', are increasingly asserting themselves (Fox *et al.*, 2005; Jouet *et al.*, 2010).

In addition to the socio-economic factors, which are the principle focus of many studies on recourse to self-medication, there are other dimensions that can also explain it: cognitive, symbolic and political. This study has brought to the forefront the mechanisms at work during the various stages of the practice.

It was however appropriate, first and foremost, to sketch, if not the whole political, economic and cultural picture, at least the context in which self-medication is practiced today. To do this, I chose to situate self-medication in the public debate it provokes, by addressing the issue of open access to medicines. In connection with the public debate on self-medication, this issue has been the object of much controversy among the actors concerned. It engenders a taking of positions by the public authorities, industry, doctors, pharmacists and users, whose stakes and logics have been examined. The actors all resort to arguments based – although in very different ways – on a rhetoric of responsibility and autonomy, of which I have demonstrated the meaning, scope and limits.

I investigated the conditions in which the subjects identify a bodily manifestation to be pathological, and the conditions in which they decide to self-medicate when confronted with what they consider to be a symptom. This reflection led me to examine the different phases through which subjects choosing to self-medicate pass: clinical self-examination, self-diagnosis and self-medication. On this point, I showed that the distinction made in medical semiology between 'objective' signs and 'subjective' signs is not operational in the framework of self-medication. We also saw that the medicalisation of a bodily sign on which the construction or identification of a symptom is based gives rise to the attribution of either an absolute value or a relative value to this symptom, and that it is this distinction between *symptoms with an absolute value* and *symptoms with a relative value* that drives the choice to take recourse to self-medication and dictates the modalities of its practice.

To delineate the motivations and the conditions for recourse to self-medication resulting from the identification of a symptom, I identified, using examples of concrete situations, four models to describe how the link between symptom identification and self-medication is formed: an empirical model, a moral model, a cognitive model and a substitutive model. Although the medical recommendations, as well as the messages accompanying the public policies, place a condition that self-medication should be limited to benign situations, we have seen that a semantic shift can take place from known *symptoms* to known *medicines* on one hand, and from *known* medicines to *benign* medicines on the other.

Moreover, the 'knowledge' of a medicine or the 'benign' nature of the situations in which the subjects are encouraged to practice self-medication far from exhaust the reasons for which they may effectively choose this recourse. Beyond the practical and economic aspects, there exist various other reasons for this practice. Indeed, we have seen that recourse to self-medication is not limited to treating benign pathologies and thereby saving on a medical consultation which is costly in time and potentially in money.

I presented recourse to self-medication within the perspective of the subjects' past experiences in order to investigate their meaning. Although, according to a commonly held belief, it is the failure to overcome a bothersome or painful symptom through self-medication that leads to a consultation with a doctor, we have seen that it is sometimes the opposite that takes place since it is a former unsuccessful recourse to a doctor (for the same symptom or a different one) that can lead to the decision to self-medicate. This case in point shows the degree to which the relationship with the medical institution is implicated in recourse to self-medication. It can thus sometimes correspond to an attempt to bypass GPs, equivalent to an evasion strategy. The decision to take such a path stems from the category of judging or critically examining medical work, since it is the doubts the patients harbour as regards their GP's competence that lead them to practice self-medication. This solution is then perceived as a substitute for a more compli-cated recourse (which may be more difficult to access, financially and practically) to a specialist doctor, or for a consultation with several GPs which could result in accusations of medical nomadism. However, recourse to self-medication, seen as an alternative to a medical consultation thought to be useless or dangerous, leads the subjects to self-medicate in situations that are not necessarily benign, with medicines that are not necessarily known. Thus a parallel is formed where the professionals disapprove of self-medication because of what they judge to be the *users'* incompetence, while the users decide on this recourse partly because of what they judge to be the *doctors'* incompetence.

In anthropology, it goes without saying that a simple reference to social rules does not suffice in accounting for behaviours (Nichter, 1989); the circumstances in which these rules are followed or broken must also be examined. From this point of view, the transformations undergone in the practice of self-medication and in its rules are inseparable from the changing (political and cultural) context in which they have been observed. Instead of the discrepancy that existed in the past between discourse and practice regarding self-medication (in other words between the discourse of dissimulation and actual practice), we now have a discrepancy between the stated conditions and the real motivations of this recourse (between benign situations and doctor avoidance strategies).

The issue of user competence is one of the major stakes on which the self-medi-cation controversy is hinged, exacerbated by the introduction of open access. This issue was examined through the question of how user knowledge is constituted. Knowledge is a fundamental stake (Rabeharisoa, 2008) both in the social debate on the competence of users and in their recourse to this practice. I have thus looked at the way the subjects' knowledge is constituted and extended, and underlined the pitfalls of this process. I showed that the mechanisms at work in self-medi-cation result from a combination of the personal work undertaken in translating a sign into a symptom (and a medicinal use into a remedy for this symptom) and the application of medical notions, acquired during previous consultations, from pharmacists or on the Internet, which are then reappropriated or reinterpreted. The practice of self-medication relies on an assessment of medicines, formed both from the knowledge the subjects have acquired from health professionals and pharmaceutical industry (Nichter and Vuckovic, 1994; Rose, 2006; Lakoff, 2006) or gained through their own experiences, and from the representations of the medicines where the symbolic logics sometimes bypass pharmacological logics.

Some of the strategies used in order to reduce the risks and increase the efficacy of drugs taken as self-medication are analogous, as we have seen, to those used for prescribed medicines, making self-medication a practice in some ways comparable to what the doctors deem to be poor compliance. Just as non-compliance can result from scepticism of a medical prescription (Conrad, 1987; Trostle, 1988; Whyte *et al.*, 2002), the act of self-medication can express a sceptical posture, or even a criticism of medical activity. Of course, not taking prescribed medicines because they are thought to have a negative or undesirable action on the body (Britten, 1996), or choosing to self-medicate and making one's own decision as to the medicines to take and the conditions in which to take them, are always affirmations of one's autonomy, even though what is expected of the subjects, in their role as autonomous beings, is above all to conform to the opinions of pharmacists, even doctors, so as to reinforce their compliance. However, it appears necessary to distinguish between self-medication and non-compliance. Because while non-compliance refers to the fact of modifying, ignoring or rejecting a treatment resulting from a *prescription*, self-medication implies a *self-prescription*. With self-medication, the subjects define the contents and modalities of their treatment themselves. While both non-compliance and self-medication involve a personal decision, the former adjusts the doctor's act of prescribing while the latter replaces it entirely. This is a meaningful difference, where what is played out is the enactment of autonomy.

The risk contained in self-medication (Fainzang, 2014), as evoked by its detractors, forms a central part of the growing debate on this practice in the public space. I have shown that the subjects develop a certain number of measures, even strategies, aiming to reduce the risks inherent in the intake of medicines (Etkin, 1992), perceived as risks in *themselves* and risks *for oneself*. I also examined the strategies aiming to maximise treatment efficacy. Ultimately, deciphering the logics that underpin self-medication shows that the practice is conceived as a means of resolving a phenomenon through the application of a balancing principle, dosing efficacy and risk, added to which the subjects implement validation techniques. We have seen in this regard that the logics used by the subjects, as irrational and estranged from biomedical logic as they may be, borrow from this medical logic, or even fed from medical notions to formulate personal, idiosyncratic (diagnostic and therapeutic) strategies, answering notably to the need to 'personalise' the treatments.

In the domain of self-medication as in other areas, health inequalities are ever present and have pernicious consequences as much on the modalities of the practice as on its effects. This is, on one hand, because the constitution of knowledge on which the practice is based is fed by variable sources, and, on the other hand, because it is realised by means of unequal material and cognitive tools.

Finally, as much through an examination of the arguments formed in the public controversy on open access, as through the recommendations linked to the practice of self-medication in the discourse of the public authorities and health professionals, I have shown that the incitation to this recourse is peppered with recommendations that empty the notion of autonomy of its contents. I will return to this point further on.

Self-medication and 'self-medicalisation'

The medicalisation of the social is a phenomenon that has been widely demonstrated in the social sciences (see for instance Conrad and Schneider, 1985; Aïach and Delanoë, 1998; Rose, 2007; Berlivet, 2011). This notion was originally used to describe the extension of the medical jurisdiction into individual life. The concept was thus understood as the medical management of a phenomenon which could be – and in the past was – managed differently, by religion or law for example (Zola, 1972). Such an understanding in fact partly reiterates the observations of functionalist authors such as Hallowell (1941) and Ackerknecht (1946) regarding the role of medicine in traditional societies.

Subsequently, medicalisation was defined more precisely as the process in which aspects of existence formerly placed outside of medical authority have come to be construed as medical problems (Conrad, 1992, 2007). The impact of medicalisation on the life of individuals is a subject of constant interest in the social sciences. Sociologists generally study medicalisation from the angle of the social control involved in transferring behaviours judged to be deviant to the medical sphere. For Conrad (2007), medicalisation occurs once a problem is defined in medical terms, described using medical language, understood through the adoption of a medical framework or treated by a medical intervention. This notion was also widely employed to describe the process by which the events of daily life fall under the influence, supervision and domination of medicine. This process was highlighted by authors such as Illich (1975) and Foucault (1988), although, according to Lupton (1997), Foucault used it a bit differently since he employed the term chiefly to emphasise how the state and medical authorities rule individuals by governing their health and their bodies. However, as Rose (2007) rightly put it, nowadays, the power of doctors is constrained by the shadow of the law, the apparatus of bioethics, evidence-based medicine, and patients' demands for autonomy to be respected, so that the focus of critique has turned to the methods used by drug companies in search of markets and profits. This notion is thus also mobilised to account for the specific role the pharmaceutical industry plays, through its incitation to treat, manage or resolve bodily or social phenomena with medicines. It is studied more and more from the angle of the fabrication of diseases by the pharmaceutical industry (Blecht, 2005) eager to create new markets, equivalent to the medical exploitation of the hazards of daily life.

The sociological and political significance of this concept resides in the fact that medicalisation – be this 'bio-medicalisation' (Clarke *et al.*, 2003), meaning a medicalisation achieved by the intervention of highly techno-scientific biomedical practices – describes a process in which non-medical problems are defined and treated as medical problems, i.e. as diseases and disorders, whether these problems have a biological foundation or not. Medicalisation is thus generally perceived as a means of intruding into individuals' lives, consisting of providing a medical response to their difficulties. A large amount of literature has endeavoured to demonstrate the medicalisation of behaviours and, more generally, of existence itself.

In this context, social scientists particularly criticise the current tendency in medicine to take an exclusively medicinal approach to human phenomena, and notably to mental suffering, which defines mental illness as something that can be relieved by a molecule (Gori & Del Volgo, 2005). Medicine – here psychiatry – responds to the commercial demands of the pharmaceutical industry, limiting itself to prescribing psychoactive drugs to contain 'deviance' and other 'behavioural troubles'. In this regard, Nichter (1989) used the term 'pharmaceuticalization' to describe 'the appropriation of human problems to medicines' (p. 272), which various French-speaking authors have echoed with the notion of '*médicamentalisation*'[3] (Desclaux and Levy, 2003) then of '*pharmaceuticalisation*' (Desclaux and Egrot, 2015), while Dumit and Greenslit (2006) evoked the 'pharmaceuticalization of culture' to account for the process by which pharmaceutical language contributes to the construction of the modern identity.

Medicalisation consists of biologising phenomena labelled as illnesses. It was thus widely used to denote the social control that results from it, of which health professionals have become the agents. What is condemned is the fact that with medicalisation there is both a dissimulation of the historical, social and political conditions that contribute to disease and suffering, and a threat to individual autonomy.[4]

However, the 'social construction' implied in the process of medicalisation cannot solely be attributed to members of the medical body and the paternity of this medicalisation is not only incumbent on health professionals. The medicalisation is no more solely down to professional authorities than the medical use of a substance is solely the result of prescriptions. It is sometimes also done by the individuals themselves, revealing not simply a medicalisation *involving* the lay world (Lowenberg and Davis, 1994; Fassin, 1998) but a medicalisation *by* the lay world. If we accept that medicalisation is the result of a social construction in that it consists of defining a problem or a phenomenon in medical language, then this construction can just as well be the work of the individuals themselves. The fact of going to the doctor's to solve a phenomenon thought to be problematic is a step that already means the person is medicalising the problem. The decision to consult one's doctor, and to thus submit to a medical judgement, participates in a process of medicalisation, which may be confirmed, prolonged or interrupted by the doctor, depending on the semiological reading he or she makes of the subject's bodily sign. In deciding to 'pathologise' a behavioural trait or a bodily manifestation by the very recourse to a medical consultation, the subject is therefore already undertaking a medicalisation of the phenomenon.

We should then recognise that not only do the subjects participate in medicalisation as soon as they decide to take recourse to a medical institution, but they are also the authors of it when they take recourse to medicines under their own initiative. Indeed, this process is down to the subjects alone when they self-medicate since they do not simply look to the expertise of a professional to confirm or reject the medical nature of the phenomenon; they provide on their own accord (be this under the influence of people around them, the Internet, etc.) a response to the problem by undergoing a medicinal treatment.

Here, I propose the term 'self-medicalisation' to describe the act of deciding for oneself to turn a given situation into a problem to be treated medically and on the strategy undertaken to tackle it (including self-information, self-governance, clinical self-examination, self-prescription, self-medication). Self-medicalisation refers to the personal decision to medicalise a problem or a phenomenon, and therefore to the belief that this problem or phenomenon should be treated. Self-medicalisation involves pathologising a behavioural trait[5] or a bodily manifestation[6] – potentially without, or against, medical opinion – and in doing so placing a situation under the medical jurisdiction that would not necessarily be there. Self-medicalisation is thus consubstantial to self-medication. When they become the sole instigator of this process, choosing alone to translate a bodily phenomenon into medical terms, and *a fortiori* when they do not merely replicate a previous prescription for an identical phenomenon, the subjects thus undertake an autonomous form of medicalisation. The individual *decision* to take psychoactive drugs to overcome sleeping difficulties or Viagra to compensate for erectile impairment is self-medicalisation before it is even self-medication. *Self-medication is the enactment of self-medicalisation.*

While the link established in the social sciences between medicalisation and social control is intended to emphasise the 'individualisation' of the social problems involved since medicalisation is said to turn a social problem into an individual one, self-medicalisation (or the medicalisation the subjects themselves undertake, potentially in opposition to or in discordance with the medical discourse) can inversely consist of turning an individual problem into a social one, through the diagnosis they make and the etiology they propose. There, self-medicalisation can equate to a politicisation of the biological phenomenon in question, even if the subject then tries to obtain a validation of the diagnosis and the therapeutic approach chosen from a professional.[7] This is the case for some of the situations described, such as when Jean-Pierre takes antihistamines to treat a cold he thinks is the result of an allergy linked to pollution, or when Edith takes anxiolytics to overcome her sleeping troubles, which she attributes to an electromagnetic field created by the proximity of a high-voltage power line, or again when Marie takes anti-inflammatories to treat her headache which she puts down to 'stress at work'. The decision to resolve a condition perceived as a problem or a disorder with medicines then validates the subject's etiology and becomes an action with social significance. While the political stake of the notion of 'medicalisation' lies, as we have seen, in emphasising a process involving the consideration of phenomena as medical when they are not necessarily, the political stake of 'self-medicalisation' leading to self-medication is to express a criticism of the structural conditions (social, economic, political) that give the bodily phenomenon in question its pathological character. In this case, there is not simply an interiorisation of medical and therapeutic perspectives (Furedi, 2006) but the assertion of both a personal judgement – although socially constructed – on one's problem and of a political act.[8]

Self-medication and autonomy

On completing this study, what can we now say about autonomy and its social treatment within the framework of self-medication? Many works have focussed on the issue of autonomy in the field of health. According to Ehrenberg (2004), we are today witnessing a 'great reversal' of the rules of contemporary individual-ity in the mental health domain, characterised by the promotion of autonomy, by individual responsibility and by the valorisation of individual initiative taking.[9] However, can this be said for other domains as well? Can we consider indeed that individual initiative is really valorised in the context of pharmaceutical self-management of a health problem? Henri Bergeron (2007) said that the process of 'autonomising' or empowering a person and his/her progressive emancipation from medical supervision leads to the development, in parallel, of a regulation of private and collective life through prevention messages. This phenomenon led him to note that what is given in individual autonomy is then taken back in social control. For other authors, the injunction to be autonomous is a trap. This goes for Massé (1999a) who asked whether, with its projects aiming to promote autonomy, the State is not attempting to shirk its responsibilities.

The issue of autonomy in medicine engages ethical positions, which result in its defenders either advocating the *right* to autonomy or the *duty* of autonomy. Carl E. Schneider (1998) thus discerned two models: the 'optional' model (which is characterised by a reluctance to believe that individuals must exercise their autonomy and an acceptance of the fact that they can, for their own reasons, not want to exer-cise it), and the 'obligatory' model (according to which it is in the patients' interests to exercise their autonomy and that they are in fact obliged to do so). Applied to the domain of self-medication however, the debate appears paradoxical. On one hand, the debate about whether autonomy should be an obligatory undertaking or an optional one is inappropriate here since self-medication itself already involves the exercise of autonomy. On the other hand, we could consider that the obligation or the recommen-dation to practice a self-medication that conscientiously follows the public authori-ties' instructions is more a case of heteronomy than autonomy, since it is then the result of a political, economic incitement from the outside and it is within this insti-tutional incitement that the principle of its action is supposed to lie. Recommending self-medication, as the public authorities do, would then be an obstacle to authentic autonomy. Rather than deciding whether autonomy should be optional or obligatory, here we should highlight the vacuity of or the contradiction in the discourse on patient autonomy where the patient is denied the real means of emancipation from medical tutelage, i.e. education and information (Fainzang, 2015). Since self-medication is a practice that exists *de facto*, patient information is all the more necessary since its absence amplifies social inequalities in access to care.

The process of 'autonomisation' and empowerment is supposed to guarantee a progressive emancipation from medical authority. Self-medication thus relates to the issue of individual liberty since, at least classically, self-medication and autonomy are closely tied to the notion of the individual. Indeed, autonomy is not generally conceived otherwise than as bound to the singular entity of a human being, at least in our societies. In this regard, the notion of autonomy does not mean the same thing in Asia as it does in the West. Macklin (1999) thus evoked cultural configurations that, while intended to protect autonomy, are not in fact rooted in the cultural value of individualism. This applies in societies where autonomy consists of family determination and not individual self-determination: in Southeast Asia, it is the family that constitutes an autonomous social unit and the doctor cannot act against that (Fan, 1997). This is why it appears necessary to distinguish here between self-medication and 'family medication', so as to avoid obliterating the often individual dimension that characterises self-medication in the West. This can lead subjects to manage their symptoms alone, unbeknown to the family and away from their prying eyes, although we should acknowledge that these practices can also sometimes consist of individuals, as we have seen, think-ing *with their family* about how to manage their affliction.

But how does this 'autonomous individual' coincide with the subject practicing self-medication? And, when the public and professional authorities recommend autonomy, do they not restrict it at the same time? The practice of self-medication does indeed presuppose the exercise of autonomy. It contains in fact all its ingre-dients if we refer to Gillon (1985) for whom autonomy is defined as the capac-ity to think and decide, and then act, freely and independently, on the basis of this thought and this decision.[10] As an avatar of autonomous conduct, self-medication is hinged on notions of 'liberty' (political, ethical and practical) and 'responsibility'. However, the public measures that encourage individual empow-erment and autonomy through the promotion of self-medication go cheek by jowl with the measures that retract them.

Today, the new users are declared to be, as we have seen, 'responsible', 'competent' and 'actors in their health'. Yet, under close examination of the mean-ing behind the public recommendations, it seems that the competence recognised in the users is limited, in the context of self-medication, to that of knowing when to self-administer a therapy recommended by a pharmacist or a doctor. The guidance about self-medication firmly excludes recourse to the domestic phar-macy (the medicine cabinet present in the subjects' homes) and tells ill people to systematically discuss the problem with a pharmacist. The demonisation of the use of a family pharmacy, based on the claim that the 'patients' are incapable of knowing how to use it wisely, goes against the recognition of their competence which is nevertheless inherent to the promotion of their autonomy.

In this regard, I have shown that the public authorities raise the spectre of the domestic pharmacy and that their discourse relating to its use limits the power of the subjects practicing self-medication. The instructions that accompany self-medication – always ask for 'advice' (and we have looked at the great ambiguity of this notion) from a pharmacist, or a doctor; never decide on a treatment on one's own; never take recourse to the family medicine cabinet – resemble the instructions regarding compliance, only differing from the strict application of pharmacist's or doctor's advice by having to pay oneself for the purchase in question. Ultimately, with self-medication, it appears that the patients should not act in accordance with their own laws, which they would not be competent to do, but they should instead simply carry out the professionals' laws in their own space. Therefore, we could wonder whether the development of self-medication is truly accompanied by an increasing *empowerment* of individuals as Blenkinsopp and Bradley (1996) postulated.

Consequently, although self-medication is supposed to respond to the need to 'give responsibility' to individuals, to their 'ability' to 'take their health in hand', to their 'capacity' to take charge of benign situations without systematically consulting a doctor, and to their desire to be 'actors in their health', the conceptual and political framework in which self-medication is defined hints at the limits to the autonomy associated with it. Although the recommendation to self-medicate is connected to a discourse on the responsible, competent, autonomous individual, the social treatment of this notion aims to turn patients into consumers who pay for their own health expenses but without for all that acknowledging their capability to make appropriate decisions. Under these circumstances, it seems that good behaviour in users involves being not too autonomous.

While the public authorities and the medical body claim to support the value of autonomy, paradoxically, self-medication, which is one of its expressions, remains deviant (and as such disapproved) as soon as it involves the ill person genuinely expressing their autonomy. The notion of autonomy is thus emptied of its contents. In these conditions, the subjects' autonomy, glorified in the promotion of self-medication, appears a mere pipe dream.

Finally, the practice of self-medication provides us with information on the relationship some users have with doctors. Indeed, played out through this practice is a relationship with the body, with medicines and with the representatives of the medical institution. It could appear paradoxical to evoke, when discussing this practice, the relationship with the medical institution in that self-medication involves forgoing it altogether. But the paradox is only in appearance since it is precisely the fact of refusing to take recourse to the medical institution that partly forms the basis of this practice, entailing a certain relationship with the health professionals that represent it. On this point, the political dimension contained in the practice of self-medication should be emphasised in so much as the practice implies a means of managing one's autonomy, and therefore one's choices, bringing into play a way of positioning oneself in the face of the public and medical authorities. With self-medication, there is a rupture in dependence on doctors, and even more so because, as we have seen, self-medication can be rooted in the desire to avoid consulting one's GP. The question of knowing the conditions in which subjects believe it appropriate to treat themselves relates to this rupture in dependence on medical authority. Although this is not necessarily equivalent to questioning the institution itself, it can consist of questioning the holder of the medical authority. Recourse to self-medication, as a therapeutic act, is thus not simply a practical or technical decision; it is also a political act, through which the subjects affirm their autonomy and their competence, which go way beyond what is granted them by the political or professional institutions.

Notes

1 The contents of which in fact differ depending on the website consulted, notably agoraforum and eurekasante, etc. [http://agoraforum.positifforum.com/t27-les-10-commandements-de-l-automedication; www.eurekasante.fr/medicaments/automedication/dix-commande-ments-automedication.html].
2 [www.eurekasante.fr/medicaments/automedication/dix-commandements-automedication.html].
3 A neologism equivalent to 'medicinisation'.
4 Lock and Nguyen (2010) qualify this claim by showing that medical practices have the possibility of simultaneously acting as a means of social control and a means of eliminating a pain or an illness, and that as such, they have the power to both subordinate and emancipate individuals.
5 For example her son's 'excitation' at bedtime which a mother tried to manage by giving him codeine for its sedative properties.
6 For example the 'sweaty hand problem' that a subject tried to control by taking an anxiolytic.
7 As suggested by the case of people who claim to be allergic, in disagreement with the medical diagnosis (Raffaetà, 2011).
8 For a more detailed presentation of this reflection, see Fainzang (2013).
9 Cited by Collin *et al.*, 2006.
10 With the reservations we have raised concerning the notion of independence.

References

Ackerknecht E.H., 1946, 'Natural diseases and rational treatment in primitive medicine', *Bulletin of the History of Medicine*, 19: 467–497.
Aïach P. and Delanoë D. (eds), 1998, *L'ère de la médicalisation*, Paris: Economica, 15–36.
Baszanger I., 2010, 'Une autonomie incertaine : les malades et le système de soins', in: E. Hirsch, *Traité de bioéthique, II. Soigner la personne, évolutions, innovations thérapeutiques*, Toulouse, Erès, 189–198.
Bergeron H., 2007, 'Les transformations du 'colloque singulier' médecin/patient: quelques perspectives sociologiques', Colloque Chaire Santé de Sciences Po / Collectif interas-sociatif sur la Santé sur: *Les droits des malades et des usagers du système de santé, une législature plus tard*, 10 p. [www.cso.edu/upload/pdf_actualites/bergeron-colloque-mars2007.pdf].
Berlivet L., 2011, 'Médicalisation', *Genèses*, 1, 82: 2–6.
Blech J., 2005, *Les inventeurs de maladies. Manœuvres et manipulations de l'industrie pharmaceutique*. Paris: Actes Sud (Babel).
Blenkinsopp A. and Bradley C., 'Patients, society and the increase of self-medication', *BMJ*, 1996, 312: 629–632.
Britten N., 1996, 'Lay views of drugs and medicines: orthodox and unorthodox accounts', in: S.J. Williams, and M. Calnan (eds), *Modern medicine. Lay perspectives and experiences*, London: UCL Press.

CCNE, 2005, 'Refus de traitement et autonomie de la personne', *Les Cahiers du CCNE*, 44: 4–23.

Clarke A.E., Mamo L., Fishman J.R., Shim J.K. and Fosket J.R., 2003, 'Biomedicalization: technoscientific transformations of health, illness and US biomedicine', *American Sociological Review*, 68, 2: 161–194.

Collin J., Otero M. and Monnais L., 2006, 'Le médicament entre science, norme et culture', in: J. Collin, M. Otero and L. Monnais (eds), *Le médicament au coeur de la socialité contemporaine. Regards croisés sur un objet complexe*, Montréal: Presses de l'université du Québec, 1–15.

Conrad P., 1987, 'The noncompliant patient in search of autonomy', *The Hastings Center Report*, 17, 4: 15–17.

Conrad P., 1992, 'Medicalization and social control', *Annual Review of Sociology*, 18: 209–232.

Conrad P., 2007, *The medicalization of society. On the transformation of human conditions into treatable disorders*. Baltimore: The Johns Hopkins University Press.

Conrad P. and Schneider J.W., 1985, *Deviance and medicalization. From badness to sickness*, Columbus: Merrill Publishing Co.

Desclaux A. and Egrot M. (eds), 2015, *Anthropologie du médicament au Sud: la pharmaceuticalisation à ses marges*, Marseille/Paris: IRD/L'Harmattan (Coll. 'Anthropologies et Médecines').

Desclaux A. and Lévy J.J., 2003, 'Cultures et médicaments. Ancien objet ou nouveau courant en anthropologie médicale?', *Anthropologie et Sociétés*, 27, 2: 5–21.

Dumit J. and Greenslit N., 2006, 'Informed health and ethical identity management', *Culture, Medicine and Psychiatry*, 30, 2: 127–134 (special issue: 'Pharmaceutical Cultures').

Ehrenberg A., 2009, 'L'autonomie n'est pas un problème d'environnement, ou pourquoi il ne faut pas confondre interlocution et institution', in: M. Jouan and S. Laugier, *Comment penser l'autonomie? Entre compétences et dépendances*, Paris: PUF (Éthique et philosophie morale), 219–235.

Ehrenberg A., 2004, 'Les changements de la relation normal-pathologique: à propos de la souffrance psychique et de la santé mentale', *Esprit*, 304, 133–155.

Etkin N.L., 1992, '"Side effects": cultural constructions and reinterpretations of western pharmaceuticals', *Medical Anthropology Quarterly* 6, 2: 99–113.

Fainzang S., 2001, *Médicaments et société. Le patient, le médecin et l'ordonnance*, Paris: Presses Universitaires de France.

Fainzang S., 2013, 'The other side of medicalization: self-medicalization and self-medication', *Culture, Medicine, and Psychiatry*, 37, 3: 488–504.

Fainzang S., 2014, 'Managing medicinal risks in self-medication', *Drug Safety*, 37, 5: 333–342.

Fainzang S., 2015, *An anthropology of lying: information in the doctor-patient relationship*, Farnham: Ashgate.

Fan R., 1997, 'Self-determination versus family determination: two incommensurable principles of autonomy', *Bioethics*, 11: 309–22.

Fassin D., 1998, 'Avant-propos : les politiques de la médicalisation', in: P. Aïach and D. Delanoe (eds), *L'ère de la médicalisation*, Paris: Anthropos/Economica, 1–13.

Foucault M., 1963, *Naissance de la Clinique. Une archéologie du regard médical*, Paris: Presses Universitaires de France.

Foucault M., 1988, Histoire de la médicalisation, Hermès, La Revue, 2, 2: 11–29.

Fox N.J., Ward K.J., O'Rourke A.J., 2005, 'The "expert patient": empowerment or medical dominance? The case of weight loss, pharmaceutical drugs and the Internet', *Social Science & Medicine*, 60, 6: 1299–1309.

Freidson E., 1984, *La profession médicale*. Paris: Payot ('Médecine et sociétés').

Furedi F., 2006, 'The end of professional dominance', *Society*, 43, 6: 14–18.

Gagnon E., 1995, 'Autonomie, normes de santé et individualité', in: J.F. Côté, (ed.), *Individualismes et individualités*, Sillery, Montreal: Septentrion, 165–176.

Gagnon E., 1998, 'L'avènement médical du sujet. Les avatars de l'autonomie en santé', *Sciences sociales et santé*, 16, 1: 49–74.

Giddens A., 1987, *La constitution de la société*, Paris: PUF.

Giddens A., 1991, *Modernity and self-identity*, Cambridge: Polity Press.

Gillon R., 1985, 'Autonomy and the principle of respect for autonomy', *BMJ*, 290: 1806–1808.

Gori R. and Del Volgo M.-J., 2005, *La Santé totalitaire: Essai sur la médicalisation de l'existence*, Paris: Denoël.

Hallowell A.I., 1941, 'The social function of anxiety in a primitive society', *American Sociological Review*, 6: 869–881.

Hoerni B., 1991, *L'autonomie en médecine. Nouvelles relations entre les personnes malades et les personnes soignantes*, Paris: Payot.

Hunter, N.D., 2010, 'Rights talk and patient subjectivity: the role of autonomy, equality and participation norms'. *Georgetown Law Faculty Publications and Other Works*. Paper 473. [http://scholarship.law.georgetown.edu/facpub/473].

Ikonomidis S. and Singer P.A., 1999, 'Autonomy, liberalism and advance care planning', *Journal of Medical Ethics*, 25, 6: 522–527

Illich I., 1975, *Némésis médicale. L'expropriation de la santé*, Paris: Le seuil.

Jouan M. and Laugier S., (eds), 2009, *Comment penser l'autonomie? Entre compétences et dépendances*, Paris: Presses universitaires de France.

Jouet E., Flora L. and Las Vergnas O., 2010, 'Contruction et reconnaissance des savoirs expérientiels des patients: Note de synthèse', *Pratiques de formation/Analyses*, 57 (special issue: 'Usagers-Experts : la part du savoir des malades dans le système de santé'): 13–94.

Lakoff A., 2006, *Pharmaceutical reason. Knowledge and value in global psychiatry*, Cambridge: Cambridge University Press (Series: Cambridge Studies in Society and the Life Sciences).

Lecomte T., 1988, 'L'automédication a-t-elle un avenir en France', *Prospective et Santé*, 47–48: 187–190.

Lecomte T., 1999, 'Chiffres de l'automédication en France et à l'étranger', in:,P. Queneau (ed.), *Automédication, autoprescription, autoconsommation*. Paris: John Libbey, 49–56.

Lock M. and Nguyen V.K., 2010, *An anthropology of biomedicine*. Malden/Oxford: Wiley-Blackwell.

Lowenberg J.S. and Davis F., 1994, 'Beyond medicalisation-demedicalisation: the case of holistic health', *Sociology of Health & Illness*, 16, 5: 579–599.

Lupton D., 1997, 'Foucault and the medicalisation critique', in: A. Petersen and R. Bunton (eds), *Foucault, health and medicine*, London: Routledge, 94–110.

Mackenzie C. and Stoljar N. (eds), 2000, *Relational autonomy: feminist perspectives on autonomy, agency, and the social self*, New York/Oxford: Oxford University Press.

Macklin, R. 1999. *Against Relativism: Cultural Diversity and the Search for Ethical Universals in Medicine*. Oxford/New York: Oxford University Press.

Marzano M., 2006, *Je consens, donc je suis... Ethique de l'autonomie*, Paris: Presses universitaires de France.

Massé R., 1999a, 'La santé publique comme nouvelle moralité', in: P. Fortin (ed.), *La réforme de la santé au Québec*, Montréal: Les Éditions Fides, 155–174.

Meyers C., 2004, Cruel choices: autonomy and critical care decision-making, *Bioethics*, 18, 2: 104–119.

Nichter M., 1989, 'Pharmaceuticals, the commodification of health, and the healthcare-medicine use transition', in: Nichter M., *Anthropology and international health. Asian case studies*, Dordrecht: Kluwer Academic Press, 265–326.

Nichter M. and Vuckovic N., 1994, 'Agenda for an anthropology of pharmaceutical practice', *Social Science and Medicine*, 39, 11: 1509–1525.

Orfali K., 2003, 'L'émergence de l'éthique clinique: politique du sujet ou nouvelle catégorie clinique?', *Sciences sociales et santé*, 21, 2: 39–70.

Pierron J.-P., 2007, 'Une nouvelle figure du patient? Les transformations contemporaines de la relation de soins', *Sciences sociales et santé*, 25, 2: 43–66.

Prayle D. and Brazier M., 1998, 'Supply of medicines: paternalism, autonomy and reality', *Journal of Medical Ethics*, 24, 2: 93–98.

Rabeharisoa V. 2008, 'Experience, knowledge and empowerment: the increasing role of patients organizations in staging, weighting and circulating experience and knowledge. State of the art', in: M. Akrich, J. Nunes, F. Paterson and V. Rabeharisoa (eds), *The dynamics of patient organizations in Europe*, Paris: Presses des Mines, 13–34.

Raffaetà R. 2011, 'The allergy epidemic, or when medicalisation is bottom-up', in: S. Fainzang and C. Haxaire (eds), *Of bodies and symptoms. Anthropological perspectives on their social and medical treatment*, Tarragona: URV Publicacions, 59–77.

Rameix S., 1997, 'Du paternalisme des soignants à l'autonomie des patients', *Laennec*, 1997, 10, 1 : 10–15.

Rose N., 2006, 'Disorders without borders? The expanding scope of psychiatric practice', *Biosocieties*, 1, 4: 465–484.

Rose N., 2007, 'Beyond medicalisation', *The Lancet*, 69, 9562: 700–702.

Rothman D.J., 2001, 'The origins and consequences of patient autonomy: a 25-year retrospective', *Health Care Analysis*, 9, 3: 255–264.

Schneewind J.B., 2001, *L'invention de l'autonomie. Une histoire de la philosophie morale moderne*, Paris: Gallimard.

Schneider C.E., 1998, *The practice of autonomy: patients, doctors, and medical decisions*, New York/Oxford: Oxford University Press.

Tristram Engelhardt H. Jr., 2001, 'The many faces of autonomy', *Health Care Analysis*, 9: 283–297.

Trostle J.A., 1988, 'Medical compliance as an ideology', *Social Science and Medicine*, 27: 1299–1308.

Whyte S.R., Van der Geest S. and Hardon H., 2002, *Social lives of medicines*, Cambridge: Cambridge University Press (coll. studies in medical anthropology).

Zola I.K., 1972, 'Medicine as an institution of social control', *Sociological Review*, 20: 487–504.

Bibliography

60 millions de consommateurs, 'La vente des médicaments en libre accès dans les pharmacies?' [www.60millions-mag.com].

Ackerknecht E.H., 1946, 'Natural diseases and rational treatment in primitive medicine', *Bulletin of the History of Medicine*, 19: 467–497.

Afipa, 2004, *Livre blanc: contribution de l'Afipa à la réflexion sur l'automédication*, Afipa document, Paris, 81 p.

Afipa, 2007, 'Pour une automédication responsable: le libre accès aux médicaments sans ordonnance en pharmacie. 1ère étape du parcours de soins du patient', doc. 27 p. [www.afipa.org/afipa/pdf/4178_afipa_communique_presse_24_oct_2007.pdf].

Aïach P., 1998, 'Les voies de la médicalisation'. in: P. Aïach and D. Delanoë (eds), *L'ère de la médicalisation*, Paris: Economica, 15–36.

Aïach P. and D. Delanoë (eds), 1998, *L'ère de la médicalisation*, Paris: Economica.

Aïach P. and Cèbe D., 1991, *Expression des symptômes et conduites de maladie*, Paris: Editions de l'Inserm/Doin.

Aïach P., Fassin D. and Saliba, J., 1994, 'Crise, pouvoir et légitimité', in P. Aïach and D. Fassin (eds), *Les métiers de la santé, enjeux de pouvoir et quête de légitimité*, Paris: Anthropos-Economica, 9–42.

Akrich A., Barthe Y. and Rémy C. (eds), 2010, *Sur la piste environnementale. Menaces sanitaires et mobilisations profanes*, Paris: Presses des Mines (coll. sciences sociales).

Akrich M., 1995, 'Petite anthropologie du médicament', *Techniques et culture*, 25–26: 129–157.

Akrich M. and Méadel C., 2002, 'Prendre ses médicaments / prendre la parole: les usages des médicaments par les patients dans les listes de discussion électroniques', *Sciences Sociales et Santé*, 20, 1 (special issue: 'Les médicaments : des prescriptions aux usages'): 89–116.

Akrich M. and Méadel C., 2004, 'Problématiser la question des usages', *Sciences Sociales et Santé* 22, 1 (special issue: 'Les technologies de l'information à l'épreuve des pratiques'): 5–20.

Alonzo A.A., 1984, 'An illness behaviour paradigm: a conceptual exploration of a situational-adaptation perspective', *Social Science and Medicine*, 19, 5: 499–510.

Anthropologie and Santé, 2011, 2, 'Anthropologie des soins non conventionnels du cancer' [http://anthropologiesante.revues.org/147].

Ardoin A.M., 1999, 'Expérience d'un pharmacien d'officine', in: P. Queneau (ed.), *Automédication, autoprescription, autoconsommation* (2ème colloque de l'APNET, déc. 1998), Paris: John Libbey, 96–100.

Aubé S. and Thoër C., 2010, 'La construction des savoirs relatifs aux médicaments sur Internet: étude exploratoire d'un forum sur les produits amaigrissants utilisés sans supervision médicale', in: Lise Renaud (ed.) *Les médias et la santé: de l'émergence à l'appropriation des normes sociales*, Coll. 'Santé et société', Québec: Presses de l'Université du Québec, 239–266.

Balcou-Debussche M., 2006, *L'éducation des malades chroniques. Une approche ethno-sociologique*, Paris : Editions des archives contemporaines.

Barbot J., 2002, *Les malades en mouvements. La médecine et la science à l'épreuve du sida*, Paris: Balland.

Barthe J.F., 1990, 'Connaissance profane des symptômes et recours thérapeutiques', *Revue française de sociologie*, XXXI, 2: 283–296.

Barthe Y., 2010, '"Cause politique et 'politique des causes". La mobilisation des vétérans des essais nucléaires français', *Politix*, 23, 91: 77–102.

Barthes R., 1972, 'Sémiologie et médecine', in: Bastide R. (ed.), *Les sciences de la folie*, Paris: Mouton, 37–46.

Barthes R., 1985, *L'aventure sémiologique*, Paris : Le Seuil.

Baszanger I., 2010, 'Une autonomie incertaine: les malades et le système de soins', in: E. Hirsch, *Traité de bioéthique, II. Soigner la personne, évolutions, innovations thérapeutiques*, Toulouse: Erès, 189–198.

Baxerres C., 2010, *Du médicament informel au médicament libéralisé. Les offres et les usages du médicament pharmaceutique industriel à Cotonou (Bénin)*, thèse EHESS/ Université Abomey-Calavi.

Beauchamp T. and Childress, J., 1979, *Principles of biomedical ethics*, New York: Oxford University Press.

Belon J.-P., 2006, *Conseils à l'officine. Aide au suivi pharmaceutique*, Paris: Masson (6th edition).

Berger P.L. and Luckmann T., 1966, *The social construction of reality: a treatise in the sociology of knowledge*, New York: Anchor.

Bergeron H., 2007, 'Les transformations du "colloque singulier" médecin/patient: quelques perspectives sociologiques', Colloque Chaire Santé de Sciences Po / Collectif interassociatif sur la Santé sur: *Les droits des malades et des usagers du système de santé, une législation plus tard*, 10 p. [www.cso.edu/upload/pdf_actualites/bergeron-colloque-mars2007.pdf].

Berlivet L, 2011, 'Médicalisation', *Genèses*, 1, 82: 2–6.

Blech J., 2005, *Les inventeurs de maladies. Manœuvres et manipulations de l'industrie pharmaceutique*. Paris: Actes Sud (Babel).

Blenkinsopp A. and Bradley C., 'Patients, society and the increase of self-medication', *BMJ*, 1996, 312: 629–632.

Bok S., 1984, *Secrets. On the ethics of concealment and revelation*. Oxford/Melbourne: Oxford University Press.

Boltanski L., 1971, 'Les usages sociaux du corps', *Annales*, 1: 205–231.

Bond C.M. and Bradley C., 1996, 'Over the counter drugs: the interface between the community pharmacist and patients', *BMJ*, 312: 758–760.

Bourdieu P., 1993, *La misère du monde*, Paris: Le Seuil, 1993.

Bret E., 2007, 'Dépendance et insuffisance respiratoire chronique', *Sciences sociales et santé*, 25, 4: 49–82.

Britten N., 1994, 'Patients' ideas about medicines. A qualitative study in a general practice population', *British Journal of General Practice*, 44, 465–468.

Britten N., 1996, 'Lay views of drugs and medicines: orthodox and unorthodox accounts', in: S.J. Williams, and M. Calnan (eds), *Modern medicine. Lay perspectives and experiences*, London: UCL Press.

Broc, C., 2003, 'La communauté des malades du sida comme fiction: les associations à l'épreuve du singulier'. *Sciences Sociales et Santé*, 3: 71–83.

Broclain D., 1994, 'La médecine générale en crise?' in: P. Aïach and D. Fassin (eds.), *Les métiers de la santé. Enjeux de pouvoir et quête de légitimité*, Paris: Anthropos, 122–160.

Brodwin P.E., 1994, 'Symptoms and social performances: the case of Diane Reden', in: M.-J. DelVecchio Good, P.E. Brodwin, B.J. Good and A. Kleinman (eds), *Pain as human experience. An anthropological perspective*, Berkeley: University of California Press, 77–99.

Buclin T. and Ammon C. (eds), 2001, *L'automédication: pratique banale, motifs complexes*, Genève: Médecine et Hygiène, Cahiers Médico-Sociaux, 11–29.

Burnier M. and Schneider M.P., 2001, 'De l'automédication à la non-observance thérapeutique', in: T. Buclin and C. Ammon (eds), *L'automédication: pratique banale, motifs complexes*, Genève: Médecine et Hygiène, Cahiers Médico-Sociaux, 89–97.

Burnier M.J. and Jeanneret O., 2001, 'L'automédication, une pratique en quête de sens: sa place dans le self care et la promotion de la santé', in: T. Buclin and C. Ammon (eds), *L'automédication: pratique banale, motifs complexes*, Genève: Médecine et Hygiène, Cahiers Médico-Sociaux, 11–29.

Callon M., Lascoumes P. and Barthe Y., 2001, *Agir dans un monde incertain. Essai sur la démocratie technique*, Paris: Le Seuil.

Calvez M., *La prévention du sida: les sciences sociales et la définition des risques*, Rennes: Presses universitaires de Rennes, 2004.

Canguilhem G., 1966, *Le normal et le pathologique*, Paris: PUF.

Cardol M., Groenewegen P.P., Spreeuwenberg P., Van Dijk L., van den Bosch W.J. and De Bakker D.H., 2006, 'Why does it run in families? Explaining family similarity in help-seeking behaviour by shared circumstances, socialisation and selection', *Soc. Sci. Med.*, 63, 4: 920–932.

Carricaburu D., Castra M. and Cohen P. (eds), 2010, *Risque et pratiques médicales*, Rennes: Presses de l'EHESP.

Cathebras P., 2000, Douleur, somatisation et culture: peut-on aller au-delà des stéréotypes? *Douleur et analgésie*, 13, 3: 159–162.

CCNE, 2005, 'Refus de traitement et autonomie de la personne', *Les Cahiers du CCNE*, 44, 4–23.

Chamberlain K., Madden H., Gabe J., Dew K. and Norris P., 2011, Forms of resistance to medications within New Zealand households, *Medische Antropologie*, 23, 2, 299–308.

Champaloux B., 2006, *Une approche anthropologique des maladies allergiques des enfants*, ATC Environnement–santé, Inserm/Ministère de la recherche, October 2006.

Charles C., Gafni A. and Whelan T., 1999, 'Decision-making in the physician-patient encounter: revisiting the shared treatment decision-making model', *Social Science and Medicine*, 49: 651–661.

Chateauraynaud F., 2002, 'Prospero, une methode d'analyse des controverses publiques', in: P. Blanchard and T. Ribémont (eds), *Méthodes et outils des sciences sociales - Innovation et renouvellement, Cahiers Politiques*, Paris: L'Harmattan, 61–84.

Chauvel L., 2006, *Les classes moyennes à la dérive*, Paris: La République des idées/Le Seuil.

Clarke A.E., Mamo L., Fishman J.R., Shim J.K. and Fosket J.R., 2003, 'Biomedicalization: technoscientific transformations of health, illness and US biomedicine', *American Sociological Review*, 68, 2: 161–194.

Collin J., 2007a, 'Relations de sens et relations de fonction: risque et médicament', *Sociologie et sociétés*, 39, 1: 99–122.

Collin J., 2007b, 'Du silence des organes au souci de soi: médicament et reconfiguration de la notion de prévention', in: I. Rossi (ed.), *Prévoir et prévoir la maladie. De la divination au pronostic*, Monts: Aux lieux d'être, 139–151.

Collin J., Otero M. and Monnais L., 2006, 'Le médicament entre science, norme et culture', in: J. Collin, M. Otero and L. Monnais (eds), *Le médicament au coeur de la socialité contemporaine. Regards croisés sur un objet complexe*, Montréal: Presses de l'université du Québec, 1–15.

Conrad P., 1987, 'The noncompliant patient in search of autonomy', *The Hastings Center Report*, 17, 4: 15–17.

Conrad P., 1992, 'Medicalization and social control', *Annual Review of Sociology*, 18: 209–232.

Conrad P., 2007, *The medicalization of society. On the transformation of human conditions into treatable disorders*. Baltimore: The Johns Hopkins University Press.

Conrad P. and Schneider J.W., 1985, *Deviance and medicalization. From badness to sickness*, Columbus: Merrill Publishing Co.

Constantinidès Y., 2008, 'Qu'est-ce que la vérité?', in: M.-F. Bacqué (ed.), *Les vérités du cancer: partager l'information, installer la relation*, Paris: Springer, 27–39.

Coulomb A. and Baumelou A., 2007, 'Situation de l'automédication en France et perspectives d'évolution: marché, comportements, positions des acteurs', Rapport établi à la demande du ministère de la santé et de la protection sociale, 32 p.

Cresson G. and Schweyer F.-X. (eds), 2000, *Les usagers du système de soins*, Rennes: Les Editions de l'ENSP.

Cresson G., 1995, *Le travail domestique de santé*, Paris: L'Harmattan.

CSA/CECOP, 2007, 'Les Français et l'automédication', enquête exclusive réalisée pour la Mutualité Française.

Dagognet F., 1996, *Pour une philosophie de la maladie*, Paris: Ed. Textuel.

DelVecchio Good M.J., Brodwin P.E., Good B.J. and Kleinman A., (eds), 1994, *Pain as human experience. An anthropological perspective*, Berkeley: University of California Press.

Deschandol P., 1998, 'Le droit des patients: le patient entre citoyen et usager', *Décision santé*, 135: 15–23.

Desclaux A. and Egrot M. (eds), 2015, *Anthropologie du médicament au Sud: la pharmaceuticalisation à ses marges*, Marseille/Paris: IRD/L'Harmattan (Coll. 'Anthropologies et Médecines').

Desclaux A. and Lévy J.J., 2003, 'Cultures et médicaments. Ancien objet ou nouveau courant en anthropologie médicale?', *Anthropologie et Sociétés*, 27, 2: 5–21.

Dew K., Chamberlain K., Hodgetts D., Norris P., Radley A. and Gabe J., 2014, Home as a hybrid centre of medication practice, *Sociology of Health & Illness*, 36, 1: 28–43.

DGS/CSA-TMO santé, 2002, *Enquête sur l'automédication*, October.

Dodds S., 2000, 'Choice and control in feminist bioethics', in: C. Mackenzie and N. Stoljar (eds), *Relational autonomy: feminist perspectives on autonomy, agency, and the social self*, New York/Oxford: Oxford University Press, 213–235.

Dodier N., 2002, 'Recomposition de la médecine dans ses rapports avec la science. Les leçons du sida', *Santé publique et sciences sociales*, 8–9: 37–52.

Dodier N., 2003, *Leçons politiques de l'épidémie de sida*, Paris: Ed. de l'EHESS.

Drulhe M., 1996, *Santé et société*, Paris: PUF.

Dumit J. and Greenslit N., 2006, 'Informed health and ethical identity management', *Culture, Medicine and Psychiatry*, 30, 2: 127–134 (special issue: 'Pharmaceutical Cultures').

Eco U., 1992, *La production des signes*. Paris: Le livre de Poche.

Ehrenberg A., 2009, 'L'autonomie n'est pas un problème d'environnement, ou pourquoi il ne faut pas confondre interlocution et institution', in: M. Jouan and S. Laugier, *Comment penser l'autonomie? Entre compétences et dépendances*, Paris: PUF (Éthique et philosophie morale), 219–235.

Ehrenberg A., 2004, 'Les changements de la relation normal-pathologique: à propos de la souffrance psychique et de la santé mentale', *Esprit*, 304: 133–155.

Emmanuel E.J. and Emmanuel L.L., 1992, 'Four models of the physician-patient relationship', *JAMA*, 267: 2221–6.

Errieau G., 1987, 'La prescription au quotidien', *Prospective et santé*, 43: 63–66.

Etkin N. L., 1992, '"Side effects": Cultural constructions and reinterpretations of western pharmaceuticals', *Medical Anthropology Quarterly*, 6, 2: 99–113.

Eugeni E., 2011, 'Living a chronic illness: a condition between care and strategies', in: S. Fainzang S. and C. Haxaire (eds), *Of bodies and symptoms. Anthropological perspectives on their social and medical treatment*, Tarragona: URV Publicacions, 111–126.

Faden R. and Beauchamp T.L., 1986, *A history and theory of informed consent*, New York: Oxford University Press.

Fainzang S., 1986, *'L'intérieur des choses'. Maladie, divination et reproduction sociale chez les Bisa du Burkina*. Paris: L'Harmattan.

Fainzang S., 1989, *Pour une anthropologie de la maladie en France. Un regard africaniste*, Paris: Ed. Ecole des Hautes Etudes en Sciences Sociales.

Fainzang S., 1996, *Ethnologie des anciens alcooliques. La liberté ou la mort*. Paris: Presses Universitaires de France.

Fainzang S., 1997, 'Les stratégies paradoxales. Réflexions sur la question de l'incohérence des conduites de malades', *Sciences Sociales et Santé*, 15, 3: 5–23.

Fainzang S., 2000, *Of malady and misery. An Africanist perspective of illness in Europe*, Amsterdam: Het Spinhuis Publishers (Coll. Health, Culture and Society).

Fainzang S., 2001a, 'Cohérence, raison et paradoxe. L'anthropologie de la maladie aux prises avec la question de la rationalité', *Ethnologies comparées*, 3. [www.academia.edu/3769107/S.Fainzang_-Coh%C3%A9rence_raison_et_paradoxe._Lanthropologie_de_la_maladie_et_la_question_de_la_rationalit%C3%A9].

Fainzang S., 2001b, *Médicaments et société. Le patient, le médecin et l'ordonnance*, Paris: Presses Universitaires de France.

Fainzang S., 2005, 'Religious attitudes toward prescriptions, medicines and doctors in France', *Culture, Medicine and Psychiatry*, 29, 4: 457–476.

Fainzang S., 2006, 'Transmission et circulation des savoirs sur les médicaments dans la relation médecin-malade', in: J. Collin, M. Otero and L. Monnais (eds), *Le médicament au coeur de la socialité contemporaine. Regards croisés sur un objet complexe*, Montréal: Presses de l'université du Québec, 267–279.

Fainzang S., 2013, 'The other side of medicalization: self-medicalization and self-medication', *Culture, Medicine, and Psychiatry*, 37, 3: 488–504.

Fainzang S., 2014, 'Managing medicinal risks in self-medication', *Drug Safety*, 37, 5: 333–342.

Fainzang S., 2015, *An anthropology of lying: information in the doctor-patient relationship*, Farnham: Ashgate.

Fan R., 1997, 'Self-determination versus family determination: two incommensurable principles of autonomy', *Bioethics*, 11: 309–22.

Fassin D., 1998, 'Avant-propos : les politiques de la médicalisation', in: P. Aïach and D. Delanoe (eds), *L'ère de la médicalisation*, Paris: Anthropos/Economica, 1–13.

Ferreira J., 1994, 'O Corpo Sígnico: uma perspectiva antropológica', in: Paulo Cesar Alves and Cecilia Souza Minayo (eds), *Saúde e Doença: um olhar antropológico*, Rio de Janeiro: Fiocruz.

Ferreira J., 2004, *Soigner les mal-soignés. Ethnologie d'un centre de soins gratuits*, Paris: L'Harmattan, Coll. Logiques sociales.

Fillion E., 2009, *A l'épreuve du sang contaminé. Pour une sociologie des affaires médicales*, Paris, Editions de l'EHESS.

Foucault J.-P., 1963, *Naissance de la Clinique. Une archéologie du regard médical*, Paris: Presses Universitaires de France.

Foucault M., 1988, Histoire de la médicalisation, *Hermès, La Revue*, 2, 2: 11–29.

Fox N.J., Ward K.J. and O'Rourke A.J., 2005, 'The 'expert patient': empowerment or medical dominance? The case of weight loss, pharmaceutical drugs and the Internet', *Social Science and Medicine*, 60, 6: 1299–1309.

Friedson E., 1984, *La profession médicale*. Paris: Payot ('Médecine et sociétés').

Furedi F., 2006, 'The end of professional dominance', *Society*, 43, 6: 14–18.

Gagnon E., 1995, 'Autonomie, normes de santé et individualité', in: J.F. Côté (ed.), *Individualismes et individualités*, Sillery, Montreal: Septentrion, 165–176.

Gagnon E., 1998, 'L'avènement médical du sujet. Les avatars de l'autonomie en santé', *Sciences sociales et santé*, 16, 1: 49–74.

Garr L., 2000, Cultural knowledge as resource in illness narratives: remembering through accounts of illness, in: C. Mattingly and L. Garro (eds). *Narrative and the cultural construction of illness and healing*, Berkeley: University of California Press.

Gautier C., 2008, 'Vers plus d'autonomie pour le patient', *Le Monde* (*Les cahiers de la compétitivité*, spécial Santé), 18 June, p. V.

Giddens A., 1987, *La constitution de la société*, Paris: PUF.

Giddens A., 1991, *Modernity and self-identity*, Cambridge: Polity Press.

Gillon R., 1985, 'Autonomy and the principle of respect for autonomy', *BMJ*, 290: 1806–1808.

Giroud J.-P., 2011, *Médicaments sans ordonnance, les bons et les mauvais*, Paris: Ed. de la Martinière.

Good B.J., 1998, *Comment faire de l'anthropologie médicale? Médecine, rationalité et vécu*. Le Plessis-Robinson: Institut synthélabo pour le progrès de la connaissance.

Good B.J. and M.-J. Delvecchio-Good, 1981, 'The meaning of symptoms: a cultural hermeneutic model for clinical practice', in: L. Eisenberg and A. Kleinman (eds), *The relevance of social science for medicine*, Dordrecht/Boston/Lancaster: D. Reidel Publishing Company, 165–196.

Gori R., Del Volgo M.-J., 2005, *La Santé totalitaire: Essai sur la médicalisation de l'existence*, Paris: Denoël.

Grand-Filaire A., 1992, 'Le bon usage du médicament en images', in *Éducation pour la santé et bon usage du médicament*, Paris: Ed. du CFES.

Guerci A., Consigliere S. and Spinelli G., 2002, 'Médicament, emballage, écriture', communication au Colloque international de l'Amades: 'Anthropologie du médicament', Aix en Provence, 21–23 March 2002.

Hagberg S., 1995, 'Cultural variations in symptom attribution', *Canadian Journal of Psychiatry*, 40, 5: 275–6.

Hallowell A.I., 1941, 'The social function of anxiety in a primitive society', *American Sociological Review*, 6: 869–881.

Hameen-Anttila K., Holappa M., Vainio K. and Ahonen R., 2010, 'What information sources do parents use when medicating their children?', proceedings of 16th International Social Pharmacy Workshop, 'Communication and information in pharmacy', Lisbonne, 23–26 August 2010.

Hamel J., 1998, 'Défense et illustration de la méthode des études de cas en sociologie et en anthropologie. Quelques notes et rappels: Figures de la connaissance', *Cahiers internationaux de sociologie*, 104: 121–138.

Hamel J., 2000, 'A propos de l'échantillon. De l'utilité de quelques mises au point', *Recherches qualitatives*, 21: 3–20.

Hammer R., 2010, *Expériences ordinaires de la médecine. Confiances, croyances et critiques profanes*, Zurich/Genève: Ed. Seismo.

Hardey M., 2001, '"E-health": the Internet and the transformation of patients into consumers and producers of health knowledge', *Information, Communication and Society*, 4, 3: 388–405.

Hardey M., 2004, 'Internet et société: reconfigurations du patient et de la médecine?", *Sciences sociales et santé*, 22, 1: 5–20.

Hassenteufel P., 1999, 'Vers le déclin du "pouvoir médical?"', *Pouvoirs*, 89: 51–64.

Haute Autorité de Santé [HAS], 2008, 'Prise en charge des médicaments soumis à réévaluation', [www.has-sante.fr].

Haxaire C., 2001, '"Calmer les nerfs": automédication, observance et dépendance à l'égard des médicaments psychotropes', *Sciences sociales et santé* (special issue : 'Les médicaments: des prescriptions aux usages'), 20, 1: 63–86.

Hay M.C., 2008, 'Reading sensations: understanding the process of distinguishing "fine" from "sick"'. *Transcultural Psychiatry*, 45, 2: 198–229.

Health Ministry (Ministère de la santé), 2008, 'Libre accès de certains médicaments devant le comptoir', Dossier Presse, 1 July [www.sante-jeunesse-sports.gouv.fr/actualite-presse/presse-sante].

Herzlich C., 1984, 'Du symptôme organique à la norme sociale', *Sciences sociales et santé*, II, 1: 11–31.

Hoerni B., 1991, *L'autonomie en médecine. Nouvelles relations entre les personnes malades et les personnes soignantes*, Paris: Payot.

Honkasalo M.-L., 1991, 'Medical symptoms: a challenge for semiotic research', *Semiotica*, 87, ¾: 251–268.

Hunter, N.D., 2010, 'Rights talk and patient subjectivity: the role of autonomy, equality and participation norms'. *Georgetown Law Faculty Publications and Other Works*. Paper 473. [http://scholarship.law.georgetown.edu/facpub/473].

Ikonomidis S. and Singer P.A., 1999, 'Autonomy, liberalism and advance care planning', *Journal of Medical Ethics*, 25, 6: 522–527.

Illich I., 1975, *Némésis médicale. L'expropriation de la santé*, Paris: Le seuil.

Institut de l'enfance et de la famille, 1994, *L'enfant, sa famille et les médicaments*, Paris: Ed. de l'Institut de l'Enfance et de la Famille.

Jaffré Y., 1999, 'La maladie et ses dispositifs', in: Y. Jaffré and J.P. Olivier de Sardan, *La construction sociale des maladies*, Paris: Les Presses universitaires de France (Collection: Les champs de la santé), 41–68.

Jonville A.-P. and Autret E., 1994, 'Les erreurs d'utilisation des médicaments en pédiatrie: étude française prospective,' in: *L'enfant, sa famille et les médicaments*, Paris: Institut de l'Enfance et de la Famille, 95–97.

Jouan M. and Laugier S., (eds), 2009, *Comment penser l'autonomie? Entre compétences et dépendances*, Paris: Presses universitaires de France.

Jouet E., Flora L. and Las Vergnas O., 2010, 'Contruction et reconnaissance des savoirs expérientiels des patients: Note de synthèse', *Pratiques de formation/Analyses*, 57 (special issue: 'Usagers-Experts : la part du savoir des malades dans le système de santé'): 13–94.

Kahneman D., 2003, 'A perspective on judgment and choice', *American Psychologist*, 58, 9: 697–720.

Karsenty S., 1994, 'L'enfant, sa famille et les médicaments: approche sociologique et anthropologique', in: *L'enfant, sa famille et les médicaments*, Paris: Institut de l'Enfance et de la Famille: 41–49.

Karsenty S., 2009, 'Le retour hétéro-déterminé de l'automédication', *Sociologie santé*, 30: 101–117.

Katz J., 1984, *The silent world of doctor and patient*, NY/London: The Free Press.

Khodoss H., 2000, 'Démocratie sanitaire et droits des usagers'. *Revue française des Affaires sociales*, 2: 111–122.

Kirmayer L.J., Young A. and Robbins J.M., 1994, 'Symptom attribution in cultural perspective', *Canadian Journal of Psychiatry*, 39, 10: 584–95.

Kleinman A., 1980, *Patients and healers in the context of culture*, Berkeley: University of California Press.

Kleinman A., 2002, 'Santé et stigmate' Note sur le danger, l'expérience morale et les sciences sociales de la santé', *Actes de la recherche en sciences sociales*, 3, 143: 97–99.

Kleinman A., Das V. and Lock M., (eds), 1997, *Social suffering*, Berkeley: University of California Press.

La Mutualité Française, 2007, 'L'Automédication: recul ou progrès?', Actes du colloque: 'Regard croisés sur l'automédication. Un colloque de la FNMF', Paris, 21 March 2007.

Lakoff A., 2006, *Pharmaceutical reason. Knowledge and value in global psychiatry*, Cambridge: Cambridge University Press (Series: Cambridge Studies in Society and the Life Sciences).

Laure P., 1998, 'Enquête sur les usagers de l'automédication: de la maladie à la performance', *Thérapie*, 53, 2: 127–135.

Le Moigne Ph., 1999, *Anxiolytiques, hypnotiques. Les facteurs sociaux de la consommation*. Document of the GDR 'Psychotropes, Politique et Société', 1.

Le Pen C., 2003, *Automédication et Santé Publique: le 'Service médical rendu' par les médicaments d'automédication*, CLP-Santé Paris, report made in collaboration with l'AFIPA.

Le Pen C., 2007, 'La consommation médicamenteuse dans 5 pays européens: une réévaluation', Paris: LEEM.

Lebeer G., 1997, La violence thérapeutique, *Sciences sociales et santé*, 15, 2: 69–98.

Lecomte T., 1994, 'La consommation pharmaceutique des enfants de moins de 10 ans d'après les données de l'enquête sur la santé et les soins médicaux réalisée en 1991–92', in: *L'enfant, sa famille et les médicaments*, Paris: Institut de l'Enfance et de la Famille, 55–68.

Lecomte T., 1988, 'L'automédication a-t-elle un avenir en France', *Prospective et Santé*, 47–48, 187–190.

Lecomte T., 1999, 'Chiffres de l'automédication en France et à l'étranger', in: P. Queneau (ed.), *Automédication, autoprescription, autoconsommation*. Paris: John Libbey, 49–56.

Légaré N., 2008, 'Les médicaments en vente libre comme substances d'abus: revue d'un phénomène méconnu', *Drogues, santé et société*, 7, 1: 129–151.

Lemorton C., 2008, 'Rapport d'information sur la prescription, la consommation et la fiscalité des medicaments', *Information report* 848, Paris: Assemblée Nationale.

Lévy J.J., 2009, 'Des essais cliniques délocalisés à l'automédication: vers une chaîne dérégulée des médicaments', in: C. Garnier and J.J. Lévy (eds), *Médicaments. De la conception à la prescription*, Montréal: Liber, 207–220.

Ligue nationale contre le cancer (1999). *Les malades prennent la parole. Le livre blanc des 1ers Etats généraux des malades du cancer.* Paris: Ramsay.

Lipovetsky G., 1992, *Le crépuscule du devoir. L'éthique indolore des nouveaux temps démocratiques*, Paris: Gallimard.

Lock M. and Nguyen V.K., 2010, *An anthropology of biomedicine*. Malden/Oxford: Wiley-Blackwell.

Lockwood G.M., 1999, 'Pregnancy, autonomy and paternalism', *Journal of Medical Ethics*, 25, 6: 537–540.

Logan K., 1983, 'The role of pharmacists and over the counter medications in the health care system of a Mexican city', *Medical Anthropology*, VII, 3: 68–89.

Low S.M., 1981, 'The meaning of nervios: a sociocultural analysis of symptom presentation in San Jose, Costa Rica', *Culture, Medicine and Psychiatry*, 5, 1: 25–47.

Lowenberg J.S. and Davis F., 1994, Beyond medicalisation-demedicalisation: the case of holistic health, *Sociology of Health and Illness*, 16, 5, 579–599.

Lupton D., 1997, 'Foucault and the medicalisation critique', in: A. Peterson and R. Bunton (eds), *Foucault, health and medicine*, London: Routledge, 94–110.

Lupton D., 2003, 'The lay perspectives on illness and disease', in: *Medicine as culture. Illness, disease and the body in western societies*. London/Thousand Oaks/New Delhi: Sage Publications.

Mackenzie C. and Stoljar N. (eds), 2000, *Relational autonomy: feminist perspectives on autonomy, agency, and the social self*, New York/Oxford: Oxford University Press.

Macklin, R. 1999. *Against Relativism: Cultural Diversity and the Search for Ethical Universals in Medicine.* Oxford/New York: Oxford University Press.

McLaughlin H., 2009, "What's in a Name: 'Client', 'Patient', 'Customer', 'Consumer', 'Expert by Experience', 'Service User'—What's Next?", *British Journal of Social Work*, 39: 1101–1117.

Martinez-Hernáez, A., 2000, *What's behind the symptom? on psychiatric observation and anthropological understanding*. Amsterdam: Harwood Academic Publishers.

Marzano M., 2006, *Je consens, donc je suis… Ethique de l'autonomie*, Paris: Presses universitaires de France.

Massé R., 1995, *Culture et santé publique*, Montréal: Gaetan Morin.

Massé R., 1997, 'Les mirages de la rationalité des systèmes ethnomédicaux', *Anthropologie et Sociétés*, 21, 1: 53–71.

Massé R., 1999a, 'La santé publique comme nouvelle moralité', in: P. Fortin (ed.), *La réforme de la santé au Québec*, Montréal: Les Éditions Fides, 155–174.

Massé R., 1999b, 'Les conditions d'une anthropologie sémiotique de la détresse psychologique', *Recherche sémiotique/Semiotic Inquiry*, 19, 1: 39–62.

Massé R., 2003, *Ethique et santé publique. Enjeux, valeurs, normativités*. Québec: Presses de l'Université Laval.

Mauss M., 1966, *Sociologie et anthropologie*, Paris: Presses universitaires de France.

McKinlay J., 1975, 'The help seeking behavior of the poor', in: J. Kosa and I. Zola (eds), *Poverty and health: a sociological analysis*, Cambridge, MA: Harvard University Press.

Mechanic D., 1980, 'The experience and reporting of common physical complaints', *Journal of Health and Social Behavior*, 21: 146–155.

Meyers C., 2004, 'Cruel choices: autonomy and critical care decision-making', *Bioethics*, 18, 2: 104–119.

Ministère de la santé, 2008, 'Libre accès de certains médicaments devant le comptoir', Dossier Presse, 1 July [www.sante-jeunesse-sports.gouv.fr/actualite-presse/presse-sante].

Mol A.-M., 2003, *The body multiple: ontology in medical practice*, Durham: Duke University Press.

Molénat X., 2010, 'De l'idéal à la norme', *Revue Sciences Humaines*, 220: 31–33.

Molina N., 1988, *L'automédication*, Paris: PUF (Coll: Les champs de la santé).

Naraindas H., 2006, 'Of spineless babies and folic acid: evidence and efficacy in biomedicine and ayurvedic medicine', *Social Science and Medicine*, 62: 2658–2669.

National Academy of Pharmacy (Académie nationale de pharmacie), 2006, 'A propos de l'automédication', rapport établi à la demande du Ministre de la santé et des solidarités, June, 26 p. [www.acadpharm.org].

Nessa J., 1996, 'About signs and symptoms: Can semiotics expand the view of clinical medicine?' *Theoretical Medicine and Bioethics*, 17, 4: 363–377.

Nichter M., 1989, 'Pharmaceuticals, the commodification of health, and the healthcare-medicine use transition', In: Nichter M., *Anthropology and international health. Asian case studies*, Dordrecht: Kluwer Academic Press, 265–326.

Nichter M. and Vuckovic N., 1994, 'Agenda for an anthropology of pharmaceutical practice', *Social Science and Medicine*, 39, 11: 1509–1525.

Nouguez E., 2007, 'Copies conformes, comportements conformes? Les patients français face au choix des médicaments génériques', *Sociologie santé*, 26 ('Système de santé et discours profanes'), 247–261.

Nylenna M. and Hjortdahl P. (1987). 'How do patients evaluate cancer related symptoms and signs? A study from general practice', *Scand J Prim Health Care*, 5: 117–122.

Orfali K., 2003, 'L'émergence de l'éthique clinique: politique du sujet ou nouvelle catégorie clinique?', *Sciences sociales et santé*, 21, 2: 39–70.

Ostermann G., 1999, 'Aspects psychologiques de l'automédication', in: P. Queneau (ed.), *Automédication, autoprescription, autoconsommation*. Paris: John Libbey, 33–38.

Oudshoorn N. and Pinch T.J. (eds), 2005, *How users matter. The co-construction of users and technology*, New Baskerville: The MIT Press.

Paicheler G., ed., 2008, 'Les femmes et le sida en France – Enjeux sociaux et de santé publique', *Médecine/Sciences*, 2: 24.

Parsons T., 1955, *Eléments pour une sociologie de l'action*, Paris: Plon, 197–238.

Peirce C.S., 1978, *Écrits sur le signe*, Paris: Seuil.

Peretti-Watel P., 2001, *La société du risque*. Paris: La Découverte, coll. Repères.

Petryna A., Lakoff A. and Kleinman A. (eds), 2006, *Global pharmaceuticals: ethics, markets, practices*, Durham: Duke University Press.

Pierret J., 1976, 'Relation au corps et conduites en maladie', *Ethnologie française*, 6: 3–4.

Pierret P., 2009, 'De l'observance à l'intégration du traitement : pour une approche dynamique', in: C. Garnier and J.J. Lévy (eds), *Médicaments, de la conception à la prescription*, Montréal: Liber, 195–205.

Pierron J.-P., 2007, 'Une nouvelle figure du patient? Les transformations contemporaines de la relation de soins', *Sciences sociales et santé*, 25, 2: 43–66.

Polillo R. and Mallet J.-O., 2007, 'Face aux professions et au management, les patients dans la redistribution des pouvoirs: éléments de comparaison en France et en Italie', in: F. Vedelago F. and M. Bouix (eds), 'Systèmes de santé and discours profanes', *Sociologie santé*, 2, 26: 175–185.

Pouchain D., Attali C., de Butler J., Clément G., Gay B., Molina J., Olombel P. and Rouy J-L., 1996, *Médecine générale. Concepts et pratique*, Paris: Masson.

Pouchelle M.-C., 2007, 'La crise de foie: une affection française?', *Terrain*, 48: 149–164.

Pouillard J., 2001, 'Risques et limites de l'automédication', *Bulletin de l'Ordre des Médecins*, April [http://bulletin.conseil-national.medecin.fr/Archives].

Pouillon J., 1977, *Fétiches sans fétichismes*. Paris: Maspero.

Prayle D. and Brazier M., 1998, 'Supply of medicines: paternalism, autonomy and reality', *Journal of Medical Ethics*, 24, 2: 93–98.

Prescrire, 2007, 'Automédication : que de confusions!', 281, March 2007.

Prescrire, 2007, *Le Guide 2008*, December, supplément au numéro 290, Tome 27.

Prescrire, 2008, 'Automédication: dire la vérité', 28, 293: 217.

Queneau P., 1999, 'Automédication en antalgiques', in: P. Queneau (ed.), *Automédication, autoprescription, autoconsommation*, Paris: John Libbey, 84–95.

Queneau P., Froudarakis M., Salvador M, Villani P. and Vital-Durand D., 2004, 'Automédication concernant les antalgiques', in: P. Queneau and G. Ostermann (eds), *Le médecin, le malade et la douleur*. Paris: Masson, 389–398.

Rabeharisoa V. 2008, 'Experience, knowledge and empowerment: the increasing role of patients organizations in staging, weighting and circulating experience and knowledge. State of the art', in: M. Akrich, J. Nunes, F. Paterson and V. Rabeharisoa (eds), *The dynamics of patient organizations in Europe*, Paris: Presses des Mines, 13–34.

Rabeharisoa V. and Callon, M., 1999, *Le pouvoir des malades. L'Association française contre les myopathies et la Recherche*. Paris: Presses de l'Ecole des mines.

Raffaetà R. 2011, 'The allergy epidemic, or when medicalisation is bottom-up', in: S. Fainzang and C. Haxaire C. (eds), *Of bodies and symptoms. Anthropological perspectives on their social and medical treatment*, Tarragona: URV Publicacions, 59–77.

Rameix S., 1997, 'Du paternalisme des soignants à l'autonomie des patients', *Laennec*, 10, 1: 10–15.

Rameix S., 1997, 'Refus de traitement et autonomie des personnes', *Pratiques*, 47: 12–15.

Raynaud D., 2008, 'Les déterminants du recours à l'automédication', *Revue Française des Affaires sociales*, 1: 81–94.

Reach G., 2007, *Pourquoi se soigne-t-on? Enquête sur la rationalité morale de l'observance*, Lormont: Editions du bord de l'eau.

Renahy E., 2008, *Recherche d'information en matière de santé sur Internet: déterminants, pratiques et impact sur la santé et le recours aux soins*, Thèse de doctorat, Université Pierre et Marie Curie.

Renahy E., Parizot I., Lesieur S. and Chauvin P., 2007, *WHIST: Enquête web sur les habitudes de recherche d'informations liées à la santé sur Internet*, Paris: Inserm U707, 20 p.

Revue Prescrire, 2008, 'Médicaments en libre accès bientôt autorisés, sûrement pas obligatoires', 28, 295: 337.

Revue Prescrire, 2012, 'Ordonnance : la dénomination commune internationale (DCI) au quotidien', 32, 346: 586–591

Rice T., 2008, 'Noisy hearts: auto-auscultation and sound in illness experience', Biennial EASA Conference: 'Experiencing diversity and mutuality', Ljubljana.

Risor M.B., 2011, 'The process of symptomization. Clinical encounters with functional disorders', in: S. Fainzang and C. Haxaire (eds), *Of bodies and symptoms. Anthropological perspectives on their social and medical treatment*, Tarragona: URV Publicacions, 21–37.

Risor M.B., 2010, 'Healing and recovery as a social process among patients with medically unexplained symptoms (MUS)', in: S. Fainzang, H.E. Hem and M.B. Risor (eds), *The taste for knowledge: medical anthropology facing medical realities*, Copenhagen: Aarhus University Press, 133–149.

Rodriguez del Barrio L. (ed), 2006, 'La gestion autonome de la médication en santé mentale. Bilan du suivi éducatif', projet pilote de collaboration entre les ressources alternatives et communautaires et le réseau public des services en santé mentale pour le renouvellement des pratiques, Erasme, Université de Montréal, 102 p.

Rogers A., 2010, 'Développer l'autogestion dans le cadre des maladies chroniques: l'exemple de l'expert patients programme (EPP)', in: I. Vincent, A. Loaec and C. Fournier (eds), *Modèles et pratiques en éducation du patient: apports internationaux*, 5è journées de la prévention, Paris, 2–3 April 2009, Saint-Denis, INPES, collection Séminaires, 121–128.

Romeyer H., 2008, 'TIC et santé: entre information médicale et information de santé', *tic et société*, 2, 1 [http://ticetsociete.revues.org/365].

Rose N., 2005, 'In search of certainty: risk management in a biological age', *Journal of Public Mental Health*, 4, 3: 14–22.

Rose N., 2006, 'Disorders without borders? The expanding scope of psychiatric practice', *Biosocieties*, 1, 4: 465–484.

Rose N., 2007, 'Beyond medicalisation', *The Lancet*, 69, 9562: 700–702.

Rothman D.J., 2001, 'The origins and consequences of patient autonomy: a 25-year retrospective', *Health Care Analysis*, 9, 3: 255–264.

Sahlins M., 1976, *Culture and practical reason*, Chicago: University of Chicago Press.

Saliba J., 1994, 'Les paradigmes des professions de santé', in: P. Aïach and D. Fassin (eds), *Les métiers de la santé. Enjeux de pouvoir et quête de légitimité*, Paris: Anthropos, 43–85.

Sand Andersen R., 2010, 'Anthropological perspectives on the biomedically defined problem of "patient delay"', in: S. Fainzang, H.E. Hem and M. B. Risor (eds), *The taste for knowledge: medical anthropology facing medical realities*, Copenhagen: Aarhus University Press, 57–68.

Sarradon-Eck A., 2007, 'Le sens de l'observance. Ethnographie des pratiques médicamenteuses de personnes hypertendues', *Sciences sociales et santé*, 25, 2: 5–36.

Sarradon-Eck A., Blanc M.A. and Faure M., 2007, 'Des usagers sceptiques face aux médicaments génériques: une approche anthropologique', *Revue d'épidémiologie et de santé publique*, 55: 179–185.

Saubadu S., 1988, *Enquête sur l'automédication: comparaison de deux groupes*, Thèse Université Paris V.

Schneewind J. B., 2001, *L'invention de l'autonomie. Une histoire de la philosophie morale moderne*, Paris: Gallimard.

Schneider C. E., 1998, *The practice of autonomy: patients, doctors, and medical decisions*, New York/Oxford: Oxford University Press.

Sebeok T.A., 1994 (1921), *Signs. An introduction to semiotics*. Toronto/Buffalo/London: University of Toronto Press.

Shands H.C., 1970, *Semiotic approaches to psychiatry*, The Hague: Mouton.

Soum-Pouyalet F., 2007, 'Le patient acteur de la thérapie et l'évolution des normes professionnelles en cancérologie', in: F. Vedelago and M. Bouix (eds), 'Systèmes de santé and discours profanes', *Sociologie santé*, 2, 26: 123–134.

Steudler F., 1999, 'Aspects sociologiques de l'automédication', in: P. Queneau (ed.), *Automédication, autoprescription, autoconsommation*. Paris: John Libbey, 23–32.

Théophile H. and Bégaud B., 2009, 'La pharmaco-épidémiologie ou l'évaluation du médicament dans la vie réelle', in: C. Garnier J.J. Lévy, editors, *Médicaments, de la conception à la prescription*, Montréal: Liber, 105–124.

Thoër C., Pierret J. and Lévy J.J., 2008, 'Quelques réflexions sur des pratiques d'utilisation des médicaments hors cadre médical', *Drogues, santé et société*, 7, 1: 19–54.

Thoër C., 2010, 'Risque médicamenteux et renégociation de la confiance au sein de la relation médecin-patient : Perspectives de médecins français et québécois sur la publication de la Women's Health initiative', *Sciences de la Société*, 76: 147–166.

Thoër-Fabre C., Garnier C., Dufort F., Levy J.J., Beaulac Baillargeon L., 2007, 'Percep-tions profanes des risques associés à l'hormonothérapie: un "bricolage" des savoirs', *Sociologie-Santé*, 26, 2 : 227–245.

Tijou Traoré A., 2010, 'L'expérience dans la production de savoirs profanes sur le diabète chez les patients diabétiques à Bamako (Mali)', *Sciences sociales et santé*, 28, 4: 41–76.

Topçu S., Cuny C. and Serrano-Velarde K., (eds), 2008, *Savoirs en débat. Perspectives franco-allemandes*, Paris: L'Harmattan.

Tourette-Turgis C., 2010, 'Savoirs de patients, savoirs de soignants. La place du sujet supposé savoir en éducation thérapeutique', *Pratiques de formation/Analyses*, 57 (special issue: 'Usagers - Experts : la part du savoir des malades dans le système de santé'): 137–153.

Trebaol E., Haxaire C. and Bail P., 2011, 'Conceptions profanes de l'usage des anti-biotiques et reception de la campagne de santé publique "les antibiotiques, c'est pas automatique"', *Sociologie Santé* (special issue: 'Les professionnels de santé: entre insti-tutions et usagers'), 33: 127–148.

Tristram Engelhardt H. Jr., 2001, 'The many faces of autonomy', *Health Care Analysis*, 9: 283–297.

Trostle J. A., 1988, 'Medical compliance as an ideology', *Social Science and Medicine*, 27: 1299–1308.

Turner V.W., 1967, *The forest of symbols, aspects of ndembu rituals*. New York: Cornell University Press.

Urfalino P., 2007, 'Médicaments et société. Enjeux contemporains. Introduction', *Annales*, 62ᵉ année, 2: 269–272.

Van der Geest S., 2010, 'Patients as co-researchers? Views and experiences in Dutch medi-cal anthropology', in: S. Fainzang, H.E. Hem and M.B. Risor (eds), *The taste for knowl-edge: medical anthropology facing medical realities*, Copenhagen: Aarhus University Press, 97–110.

Van der Geest S. and Whyte S.R., 1988, *The context of medicines in developing countries*, Dordrecht: Kluwer Academic Publishers.

Van der Geest S., S.R. Whyte and A. Hardon, 1996, 'The anthropology of pharmaceuticals: a biographical approach', *Annual Review of Anthropology*, 25: 153–178.

Vega A., 2011, 'Le partage des responsabilités en médecine. Une approche socio-anthropologique des pratiques soignantes', report for the CNAMTS, 199 p.

Vincent I., Loaec A and Fournier C. (eds), 2010, *Modèles et pratiques en éducation du patient: apports internationaux*, 5è journées de la prévention, Paris, 2–3 April 2009, Saint-Denis, INPES, collection Séminaires.

Walger O., 2009, 'Empowerment et soutien social des personnes vivant avec un diabète: développement d'un outil d'évaluation à usage clinique', *Education du Patient et Enjeux de Santé*, 27, 1: 5–12.

Wallach I., 2008, 'Automédication et pluralisme thérapeutique chez les jeunes d'origine chinoise vivant en France et au Québec', *Revue internationale sur le médicament*, 2: 139–185.

Wallach M., 2001, '"Automédication responsible": un partenariat pharmaciens-industriels pour le bienfait des consommateurs', in: T. Buclin and C. Ammon (eds), *L'automédication, pratique banale, motifs complexes*, Genève: Editions Médecine et Hygiène, 167–171.

Whyte S.R., Van der Geest S. and Hardon H., 2002, *Social lives of medicines*, Cambridge: Cambridge University Press (coll. studies in medical anthropology).

Winance M., 2007, 'Dépendance versus autonomie… de la signification et de l'imprégnation de ces notions dans les pratiques médico-sociales', *Sciences sociales et santé*, 4: 83–91.

Woolf V., 2007, *De la maladie*, Paris: Payot and Rivages.

Wyatt S., Henvood H.A. and Platzer H., 2004, 'L'extension des territoires du patient: Internet et santé au quotidien', *Sciences sociales et santé*, 1: 45–68.

Young A., 1976, 'Some implications of medical beliefs and practices for social anthropology', *American Anthropologist*, 78: 5–24.

Zborowski M., 1952, 'Cultural components in response to pain', *J Soc Issues* 8: 16–30.

Zola I.K., 1966, 'Culture and symptoms. An analysis of patients' presenting complaints', *Amer. Sociol. Rev.*, 31: 615–30.

Zola I.K., 1972, 'Medicine as an institution of social control', *Sociological Review*, 20: 487–504.

Index